C-Reactive Protein and Cardiovascular Disease: Clinical Aspects

C-Reactive Protein and Cardiovascular Disease: Clinical Aspects

Editor

Ahmed Sheriff

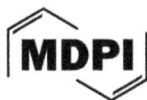

Basel • Beijing • Wuhan • Barcelona • Belgrade • Novi Sad • Cluj • Manchester

Editor
Ahmed Sheriff
Charité University Medicine
Berlin, Germany

Editorial Office
MDPI
St. Alban-Anlage 66
4052 Basel, Switzerland

This is a reprint of articles from the Special Issue published online in the open access journal *Journal of Clinical Medicine* (ISSN 2077-0383) (available at: https://www.mdpi.com/journal/jcm/special_issues/C-reactive_protein).

For citation purposes, cite each article independently as indicated on the article page online and as indicated below:

Lastname, A.A.; Lastname, B.B. Article Title. *Journal Name* **Year**, *Volume Number*, Page Range.

ISBN 978-3-0365-9943-4 (Hbk)
ISBN 978-3-0365-9944-1 (PDF)
doi.org/10.3390/books978-3-0365-9944-1

© 2024 by the authors. Articles in this book are Open Access and distributed under the Creative Commons Attribution (CC BY) license. The book as a whole is distributed by MDPI under the terms and conditions of the Creative Commons Attribution-NonCommercial-NoDerivs (CC BY-NC-ND) license.

Contents

About the Editor . . . . **vii**

Ahmed Sheriff
Special Issue "C-Reactive Protein and Cardiovascular Disease: Clinical Aspects"
Reprinted from: *J. Clin. Med.* **2022**, *11*, 3610, doi:10.3390/jcm11133610 . . . . **1**

Magdalena Holzknecht, Christina Tiller, Martin Reindl, Ivan Lechner, Priscilla Fink, Patrick Lunger, et al.
Association of C-Reactive Protein Velocity with Early Left Ventricular Dysfunction in Patients with First ST-Elevation Myocardial Infarction
Reprinted from: *J. Clin. Med.* **2021**, *10*, 5494, doi:10.3390/jcm10235494 . . . . **5**

Rafael Y. Brzezinski, Ariel Melloul, Shlomo Berliner, Ilana Goldiner, Moshe Stark, Ori Rogowski, et al.
Early Detection of Inflammation-Prone STEMI Patients Using the CRP Troponin Test (CTT)
Reprinted from: *J. Clin. Med.* **2022**, *11*, 2453, doi:10.3390/jcm11092453 . . . . **17**

Ronnie Meilik, Hadas Ben-Assayag, Ahuva Meilik, Shlomo Berliner, David Zeltser, Itzhak Shapira, et al.
Sepsis Related Mortality Associated with an Inflammatory Burst in Patients Admitting to the Department of Internal Medicine with Apparently Normal C-Reactive Protein Concentration
Reprinted from: *J. Clin. Med.* **2022**, *11*, 3151, doi:10.3390/jcm11113151 . . . . **27**

Jan Torzewski, Patrizia Brunner, Wolfgang Ries, Christoph D. Garlichs, Stefan Kayser, Franz Heigl and Ahmed Sheriff
Targeting C-Reactive Protein by Selective Apheresis in Humans: Pros and Cons
Reprinted from: *J. Clin. Med.* **2022**, *11*, 1771, doi:10.3390/jcm11071771 . . . . **37**

Fabrizio Esposito, Harald Matthes and Friedemann Schad
Seven COVID-19 Patients Treated with C-Reactive Protein (CRP) Apheresis
Reprinted from: *J. Clin. Med.* **2022**, *11*, 1956, doi:10.3390/jcm11071956 . . . . **49**

Myron Zaczkiewicz, Katharina Kostenzer, Matthias Graf, Benjamin Mayer, Oliver Zimmermann and Jan Torzewski
Cardiac Glycosides Lower C-Reactive Protein Plasma Levels in Patients with Decompensated Heart Failure: Results from the Single-Center C-Reactive Protein-Digoxin Observational Study (C-DOS)
Reprinted from: *J. Clin. Med.* **2022**, *11*, 1762, doi:10.3390/jcm11071762 . . . . **61**

Hack-Lyoung Kim, Woo-Hyun Lim, Jae-Bin Seo, Sang-Hyun Kim, Joo-Hee Zo and Myung-A Kim
Improved Prognostic Value in Predicting Long-Term Cardiovascular Events by a Combination of High-Sensitivity C-Reactive Protein and Brachial–Ankle Pulse Wave Velocity
Reprinted from: *J. Clin. Med.* **2021**, *10*, 3291, doi:10.3390/jcm10153291 . . . . **71**

Helena Enocsson, Jesper Karlsson, Hai-Yun Li, Yi Wu, Irving Kushner, Jonas Wetterö and Christopher Sjöwall
The Complex Role of C-Reactive Protein in Systemic Lupus Erythematosus
Reprinted from: *J. Clin. Med.* **2021**, *10*, 5837, doi:10.3390/jcm10245837 . . . . **81**

Karen Pesqueda-Cendejas, Isela Parra-Rojas, Paulina E. Mora-García,
Margarita Montoya-Buelna, Adolfo I. Ruiz-Ballesteros, Mónica R. Meza-Meza, et al.
CRP Serum Levels Are Associated with High Cardiometabolic Risk and Clinical Disease
Activity in Systemic Lupus Erythematosus Patients
Reprinted from: *J. Clin. Med.* **2022**, *11*, 1849, doi:10.3390/jcm11071849 . . . . **97**

Gerd Wallukat, Stephan Mattecka, Katrin Wenzel, Wieland Schrödl, Birgit Vogt,
Patrizia Brunner, et al.
C-Reactive Protein (CRP) Blocks the Desensitization of Agonistic Stimulated G Protein Coupled
Receptors (GPCRs) in Neonatal Rat Cardiomyocytes
Reprinted from: *J. Clin. Med.* **2022**, *11*, 1058, doi:10.3390/jcm11041058 . . . . **113**

About the Editor

Ahmed Sheriff

Ahmed Sheriff is a biochemist with several years of research on the immunology of inflammatory diseases at the Institute for Clinical Immunology at the University of Erlangen. Previously, Dr. Sheriff gained corporate experience in the biotechnology company Genethor GmbH, which he founded. From 2007 to 2008, Dr. Sheriff was the Managing Director of the European Federation of Immunological Societies. From 2007 to 2010, he was the Managing Director of the German Society for Immunology. In 2008, his path also led him to Charité Universitätsmedizin in Berlin, where he developed a CRP adsorber and conducted preclinical research together with the Nephrology, Intensive Care Medicine, and Cardiology departments of Charité's Virchow Clinic. In 2010, the need arose to pursue this topic further in a start-up (Pentracor GmbH), as research funding was impossible. In the meantime, a clinical study and several registries have demonstrated the positive potential of CRP apheresis in myocardial infarction, cardiogenic shock, and the severe course of COVID-19.

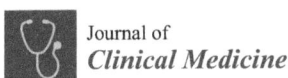

Editorial

Special Issue "C-Reactive Protein and Cardiovascular Disease: Clinical Aspects"

Ahmed Sheriff [1,2]

[1] Division of Gastroenterology, Infectiology and Rheumatology, Medical Department, Charité University Medicine, 12200 Berlin, Germany; ahmed.sheriff@charite.de
[2] Pentracor GmbH, 16761 Hennigsdorf, Germany

1. Prologue: The Prehistoric Antibody CRP and Its Immune Complexes

This Special Issue focuses on the clinical relevance of C-reactive protein. Most physicians are familiar with it as a diagnostic biomarker. Only a few have realised that it can be a pathomolecule. After all, biomarker is of course not a physiological function. The main task of CRP is to mark cells to be disposed of, which has been shown for decades in various animal models and has been broken down to the molecular detail [1,2]. For several decades, CRP has been established as an extremely sensitive, reliable and early indicator of inflammatory and tissue-destructive processes. Following an acute phase stimulus, up to 1000-fold increased values can be measured.

This prototype of the human acute phase protein has been considered an inflammatory marker since it was first described by Tillet and Francis in 1930 [3].

However, the mere use of CRP as a readily measurable inflammation marker neglects the biological function of the protein.

CRP is a serum protein and a mediator of innate immunity. The diverse functions of CRP across all living species led to the conclusion that CRP is a prehistoric precursor of all antibodies in the evolutionarily much later appearing mammals.

Already in the horseshoe crab (Limulus), a "living fossil" at least 250 million years old, CRP forms immune complexes together with complement and thus assumes defence functions. At the same time, it acts phylogenetically as an antibody in numerous species, such as fish, which have no adaptive immune system. In humans, its functions are complex and part of re-intensified research.

It is now accepted, even if not everyone is aware of it, that CRP plays a central role in the development of inflammation-related tissue damage [4]. CRP activates (like antibodies) the complement system via the classical pathway [5] and macrophages via Fc receptors [6,7]. Therefore, CRP, like antibodies, binds to Fc receptors.

2. The CRP Increase of the First 48 h

Most recently, a significant correlation of the CRP increase after myocardial infarction with the size of the damage was also shown in humans, as well as the reduction of the damage by CRP removal [2,8]. The relevance of the initial increase in CRP levels in the first approximately 48h for prognosis is described by three articles in this Special Issue [9–11]. This is confirmed by several recent articles [8,12]. This is an additional clear indication that attention should be paid to CRP in terms of pathological properties.

3. CRP Triggers the Disposal of Hypoxic and Ischaemic Cells

The findings from the removal of CRP after STEMI or in severe COVID-19 by CRP apheresis are summarised in the article by Torzewski et al. [13]. The influence of CRP in other cardiovascular disease patterns (atherosclerosis, myocarditis and dilated cardiomyopathy, stroke) and autoimmune diseases (e.g., rheumatoid arthritis, ulcerative colitis,

Crohn's disease, psoriasis, giant cell arteritis) is also discussed. It is also reported here which other drugs are/were already tried to block CRP or reduce its amount.

Very impressively, it was shown by Esposito et al. [14] how beneficial the removal of CRP is in severe COVID-19. The treatments were performed within the CACOV registry to allow for scientific evaluation. The impressive before/after CT and X-ray images of the patients' lungs speak volumes. This is a very exciting report on a poorly known treatment option for severe COVID-19. Even though it is not a clinical trial, the results are remarkable. Not only was the mortality rate very low in a patient group where >40% would have been expected, but the normally progressive damage to the lungs was also reversed. Additionally, the 50% mortality rate within 12 months of hospitalisation was not seen in this severe cohort. A case series from the same registry (CACOV) with almost the same outcome was recently reported from another hospital [15]. The report by Esposito et al. spectacularly confirms that oxygen-deprived cells get the problem of being disposed of because of CRP, and this actually does not happen when a sufficient amount of CRP is removed from the blood plasma.

The inflammation in the lungs and other tissues caused by the severe acute respiratory syndrome coronavirus 2 (SARS-CoV-2) was and is a disease with a high mortality rate, for which there were still no comprehensive, effective and approved treatment guidelines in spring 2021, but only recommendations.

Even the first publications from Wuhan and later from Italy and the USA showed that this is not an infectious disease in the classical sense, but a strongly immunologically controlled disease [16–18]. Accordingly, a deeper understanding of the specific inflammatory process is essential.

Systemic inflammation, measurable for example by C-reactive protein, is correlated with thromboembolic events, acute renal failure, severe courses, ventilation requirement and intensive care requirement, as well as high mortality and high post-discharge mortality in COVID-19 [19–21].

This increased plasma CRP level correlates inversely with prognosis in all publications published since then. This is scientific consensus. The odds ratio for mortality increases with the amount of CRP and rises dramatically to over 23 at CRP > 250 mg/L [22].

4. CRP and Heart Failure

Zaczkiewicz et al. [23] present an interesting article reporting data from a prospective observational study at a single centre—60 patients with decompensated heart failure. The aim of this study was to investigate whether CRP plasma levels could be reduced by digoxin in addition to optimal medical treatment in patients with heart failure and reduced left ventricular ejection fraction who were hospitalised with decompensated heart failure (NYHA class III and IV). The authors investigated an important issue in the heart failure population. Due to standard heart failure treatment, CRP levels were significantly lower in each group at day 21–day 1 and day 21–day 3. Comparison of the extent of CRP plasma level reduction at day 21–day 3 between the two groups showed borderline significance ($p = 0.051$). Despite the fact that statistical significance was not reached between the groups studied and the number of study participants is small, the study will add to the current knowledge in this field. This study can serve as a basis for further research.

5. CRP and Arterial Stiffness Are Associated with the Development of Cardiovascular Disease

Using data from a retrospective single-centre study, Kim and colleagues showed that elevated levels of brachial-ankle pulse wave velocity (baPWV) and C-reactive protein (CRP) were associated with serious adverse cardiovascular events (MACE), even after adjustment for covariates. Furthermore, they showed that the combination of baPWV and CRP further stratified subjects' risk. They concluded that the combination of CRP and baPWV was better at predicting future cardiovascular death than either value alone. The concepts of the study are easy to understand, and the combination of baPWV and CRP in this study has some innovations [24].

6. CRP in Systemic Lupus Erythematosus

Two articles address systemic lupus erythematosus (SLE). Both describe the cardiovascular risk as a function of the CRP concentration. This sounds a bit paradoxical, as SLE patients are characterised by their inability to synthesise high enough amounts of CRP. Allow the authors to illustrate this point for you. The review by Enocsson et al. [25] summarizes the biological effect of CRP in autoimmune conditions and additionally highlights the role of CRP for cardiovascular diseases. It also takes into account the influence of other inflammatory and/or clearance related proteins such as IL6, interferon, complement or CRP autoantigens. Pesqueda-Cendejas and colleagues [26] report that high CRP levels were connected with high cardiometabolic risk and high clinical disease activity in SLE patients. This implication is not a surprise; however, the cohorts are very well selected and consist of a large number of female patients with the same ethnicity.

7. CRP's Influence on G-Protein Coupled Receptors

In another article [27], a new, previously undescribed property of CRP is reported. CRP interferes with the desensitization of G-protein coupled receptors (GPCRs) and has to be considered as a novel regulator of adrenergic, angiotensin-1 and endothelin receptors. This is a surprise because CRP's molecular action has so far only been investigated on, e.g., Fc receptor γRII (FcγRII) and in the context of macrophage activation and its role as an archaic antibody-like molecule. In addition, CRP induces the classical complement pathway after binding to its ligand, which produces immune complexes. However, the direct influence of CRP on the cardiovascular system of rabbits has also been reported recently [28], which has nothing to do with a lack of oxygen supply. Surprisingly, the effect takes place on well energised cells. What might this mean with regard to tachycardia in high inflammation?

8. Epilogue

The articles presented in this Special Issue reveal a broad spectrum of indications with CRP involvement. The reports unanimously support the view that CRP has a dark side. In addition to this new perspective about pathological properties of CRP, two other new aspects are crystallising. One is that the initial rate of CRP synthesis in an acute illness such as sepsis or myocardial infarction allows an excellent prognosis in terms of mortality or cardiac function/scar area. The other is the surprising finding that CRP impairs the desensitisation of GPCRs without the need for any further damaging process. I am curious to learn what other features CRP has kept from us so far.

Funding: This research received no external funding.

Conflicts of Interest: The author declares no conflict of interest.

References

1. Sheriff, A.; Kayser, S.; Brunner, P.; Vogt, B. C-Reactive Protein Triggers Cell Death in Ischemic Cells. *Front. Immunol.* **2021**, *12*, 630430. [CrossRef] [PubMed]
2. Buerke, M.; Sheriff, A.; Garlichs, C.D. CRP apheresis in acute myocardial infarction and COVID-19. *Med. Klin. Intensivmed. Notf.* **2022**, *117*, 191–199. [CrossRef] [PubMed]
3. Tillett, W.S.; Francis, T. Serological Reactions in Pneumonia with a Non-Protein Somatic Fraction of Pneumococcus. *J. Exp. Med.* **1930**, *52*, 561–571. [CrossRef] [PubMed]
4. Kunze, R. C-Reactive Protein: From Biomarker to Trigger of Cell Death? *Ther. Apher. Dial.* **2019**, *23*, 494–496. [CrossRef] [PubMed]
5. Kaplan, M.H.; Volanakis, J.E. Interaction of C-reactive protein complexes with the complement system. I. Consumption of human complement associated with the reaction of C-reactive protein with pneumococcal C-polysaccharide and with the choline phosphatides, lecithin and sphingomyelin. *J. Immunol.* **1974**, *112*, 2135–2147. [PubMed]
6. Bharadwaj, D.; Stein, M.P.; Volzer, M.; Mold, C.; Du Clos, T.W. The major receptor for C-reactive protein on leukocytes is fcgamma receptor II. *J. Exp. Med.* **1999**, *190*, 585–590. [CrossRef]

7. Manolov, D.E.; Rocker, C.; Hombach, V.; Nienhaus, G.U.; Torzewski, J. Ultrasensitive confocal fluorescence microscopy of C-reactive protein interacting with FcgammaRIIa. *Arterioscler. Thromb. Vasc. Biol.* **2004**, *24*, 2372–2377. [CrossRef]
8. Ries, W.; Torzewski, J.; Heigl, F.; Pfluecke, C.; Kelle, S.; Darius, H.; Ince, H.; Mitzner, S.; Nordbeck, P.; Butter, C.; et al. C-Reactive Protein Apheresis as Anti-inflammatory Therapy in Acute Myocardial Infarction: Results of the CAMI-1 Study. *Front. Cardiovasc. Med.* **2021**, *8*, 591714. [CrossRef]
9. Holzknecht, M.; Tiller, C.; Reindl, M.; Lechner, I.; Fink, P.; Lunger, P.; Mayr, A.; Henninger, B.; Brenner, C.; Klug, G.; et al. Association of C-Reactive Protein Velocity with Early Left Ventricular Dysfunction in Patients with First ST-Elevation Myocardial Infarction. *J. Clin. Med.* **2021**, *10*, 5494. [CrossRef]
10. Brzezinski, R.Y.; Melloul, A.; Berliner, S.; Goldiner, I.; Stark, M.; Rogowski, O.; Banai, S.; Shenhar-Tsarfaty, S.; Shacham, Y. Early Detection of Inflammation-Prone STEMI Patients Using the CRP Troponin Test (CTT). *J. Clin. Med.* **2022**, *11*, 2453. [CrossRef]
11. Meilik, R.; Ben-Assayag, H.; Meilik, A.; Berliner, S.; Zeltser, D.; Shapira, I.; Rogowski, O.; Goldiner, I.; Shenhar-Tsarfaty, S.; Wasserman, A. Sepsis Related Mortality Associated with an Inflammatory Burst in Patients Admitting to the Department of Internal Medicine with Apparently Normal C-Reactive Protein Concentration. *J. Clin. Med.* **2022**, *11*, 3151. [CrossRef] [PubMed]
12. Banai, A.; Levit, D.; Morgan, S.; Loewenstein, I.; Merdler, I.; Hochstadt, A.; Szekely, Y.; Topilsky, Y.; Banai, S.; Shacham, Y. Association between C-Reactive Protein Velocity and Left Ventricular Function in Patients with ST-Elevated Myocardial Infarction. *J. Clin. Med.* **2022**, *11*, 401. [CrossRef] [PubMed]
13. Torzewski, J.; Brunner, P.; Ries, W.; Garlichs, C.D.; Kayser, S.; Heigl, F.; Sheriff, A. Targeting C-Reactive Protein by Selective Apheresis in Humans: Pros and Cons. *J. Clin. Med.* **2022**, *11*, 1771. [CrossRef]
14. Esposito, F.; Matthes, H.; Schad, F. Seven COVID-19 Patients Treated with C-Reactive Protein (CRP) Apheresis. *J. Clin. Med.* **2022**, *11*, 1956. [CrossRef] [PubMed]
15. Schumann, C.; Heigl, F.; Rohrbach, I.J.; Sheriff, A.; Wagner, L.; Wagner, F.; Torzewski, J. A Report on the First 7 Sequential Patients Treated Within the C-Reactive Protein Apheresis in COVID (CACOV) Registry. *Am. J. Case Rep.* **2022**, *23*, e935263. [CrossRef]
16. Ruan, Q.; Yang, K.; Wang, W.; Jiang, L.; Song, J. Clinical predictors of mortality due to COVID-19 based on an analysis of data of 150 patients from Wuhan, China. *Intensive Care Med.* **2020**, *46*, 846–848. [CrossRef] [PubMed]
17. Guan, W.J.; Ni, Z.Y.; Hu, Y.; Liang, W.H.; Ou, C.Q.; He, J.X.; Liu, L.; Shan, H.; Lei, C.L.; Hui, D.S.C.; et al. Clinical Characteristics of Coronavirus Disease 2019 in China. *N. Engl. J. Med.* **2020**, *382*, 1708–1720. [CrossRef]
18. Tan, C.; Huang, Y.; Shi, F.; Tan, K.; Ma, Q.; Chen, Y.; Jiang, X.; Li, X. C-reactive protein correlates with computed tomographic findings and predicts severe COVID-19 early. *J. Med. Virol.* **2020**, *92*, 856–862. [CrossRef]
19. Mueller, A.A.; Tamura, T.; Crowley, C.P.; DeGrado, J.R.; Haider, H.; Jezmir, J.L.; Keras, G.; Penn, E.H.; Massaro, A.F.; Kim, E.Y. Inflammatory Biomarker Trends Predict Respiratory Decline in COVID-19 Patients. *Cell Rep. Med.* **2020**, *1*, 100144. [CrossRef]
20. Smilowitz, N.R.; Kunichoff, D.; Garshick, M.; Shah, B.; Pillinger, M.; Hochman, J.S.; Berger, J.S. C-reactive protein and clinical outcomes in patients with COVID-19. *Eur. Heart J.* **2021**, *42*, 2270–2279. [CrossRef]
21. Gunster, C.; Busse, R.; Spoden, M.; Rombey, T.; Schillinger, G.; Hoffmann, W.; Weber-Carstens, S.; Schuppert, A.; Karagiannidis, C. 6-month mortality and readmissions of hospitalized COVID-19 patients: A nationwide cohort study of 8679 patients in Germany. *PLoS ONE* **2021**, *16*, e0255427. [CrossRef]
22. Stefan, N.; Sippel, K.; Heni, M.; Fritsche, A.; Wagner, R.; Jakob, C.E.M.; Preissl, H.; von Werder, A.; Khodamoradi, Y.; Borgmann, S.; et al. Obesity and Impaired Metabolic Health Increase Risk of COVID-19-Related Mortality in Young and Middle-Aged Adults to the Level Observed in Older People: The LEOSS Registry. *Front. Med.* **2022**, *9*, 875430. [CrossRef] [PubMed]
23. Zaczkiewicz, M.; Kostenzer, K.; Graf, M.; Mayer, B.; Zimmermann, O.; Torzewski, J. Cardiac Glycosides Lower C-Reactive Protein Plasma Levels in Patients with Decompensated Heart Failure: Results from the Single-Center C-Reactive Protein-Digoxin Observational Study (C-DOS). *J. Clin. Med.* **2022**, *11*, 1762. [CrossRef] [PubMed]
24. Kim, H.L.; Lim, W.H.; Seo, J.B.; Kim, S.H.; Zo, J.H.; Kim, M.A. Improved Prognostic Value in Predicting Long-Term Cardiovascular Events by a Combination of High-Sensitivity C-Reactive Protein and Brachial-Ankle Pulse Wave Velocity. *J. Clin. Med.* **2021**, *10*, 3291. [CrossRef] [PubMed]
25. Enocsson, H.; Karlsson, J.; Li, H.Y.; Wu, Y.; Kushner, I.; Wettero, J.; Sjowall, C. The Complex Role of C-Reactive Protein in Systemic Lupus Erythematosus. *J. Clin. Med.* **2021**, *10*, 5837. [CrossRef]
26. Pesqueda-Cendejas, K.; Parra-Rojas, I.; Mora-Garcia, P.E.; Montoya-Buelna, M.; Ruiz-Ballesteros, A.I.; Meza-Meza, M.R.; Campos-Lopez, B.; Rivera-Escoto, M.; Vizmanos-Lamotte, B.; Cerpa-Cruz, S.; et al. CRP Serum Levels Are Associated with High Cardiometabolic Risk and Clinical Disease Activity in Systemic Lupus Erythematosus Patients. *J. Clin. Med.* **2022**, *11*, 1849. [CrossRef]
27. Wallukat, G.; Mattecka, S.; Wenzel, K.; Schrodl, W.; Vogt, B.; Brunner, P.; Sheriff, A.; Kunze, R. C-Reactive Protein (CRP) Blocks the Desensitization of Agonistic Stimulated G Protein Coupled Receptors (GPCRs) in Neonatal Rat Cardiomyocytes. *J. Clin. Med.* **2022**, *11*, 1058. [CrossRef]
28. Bock, C.; Vogt, B.; Mattecka, S.; Yapici, G.; Brunner, P.; Fimpel, S.; Unger, J.K.; Sheriff, A. C-Reactive Protein Causes Blood Pressure Drop in Rabbits and Induces Intracellular Calcium Signaling. *Front. Immunol.* **2020**, *11*, 1978. [CrossRef]

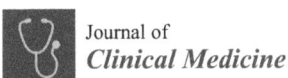

Article

Association of C-Reactive Protein Velocity with Early Left Ventricular Dysfunction in Patients with First ST-Elevation Myocardial Infarction

Magdalena Holzknecht [1], Christina Tiller [1], Martin Reindl [1], Ivan Lechner [1], Priscilla Fink [1], Patrick Lunger [1], Agnes Mayr [2], Benjamin Henninger [2], Christoph Brenner [1], Gert Klug [1], Axel Bauer [1], Bernhard Metzler [1] and Sebastian Johannes Reinstadler [1],*

[1] University Clinic of Internal Medicine III Cardiology and Angiology, Medical University of Innsbruck, Anichstrasse 35, 6020 Innsbruck, Austria; Magdalena.Holzknecht@tirol-kliniken.at (M.H.); Christina.Tiller@tirol-kliniken.at (C.T.); Martin.Reindl@tirol-kliniken.at (M.R.); Ivan.Lechner@tirol-kliniken.at (I.L.); Priscilla.Fink@tirol-kliniken.at (P.F.); Patrick.Lunger@student.i-med.ac.at (P.L.); Christoph.Brenner@tirol-kliniken.at (C.B.); Gert.Klug@tirol-kliniken.at (G.K.); Axel.Bauer@tirol-kliniken.at (A.B.); Bernhard.Metzler@tirol-kliniken.at (B.M.)
[2] University Clinic of Radiology, Medical University of Innsbruck, Anichstrasse 35, 6020 Innsbruck, Austria; A.Mayr@i-med.ac.at (A.M.); Benjamin.Henninger@tirol-kliniken.at (B.H.)
* Correspondence: Sebastian.Reinstadler@gmail.com; Tel.: +43-51250481317; Fax: +43-51250422767

Abstract: C-reactive protein velocity (CRPv) has been proposed as a very early and sensitive risk predictor in patients with ST-elevation myocardial infarction (STEMI). However, the association of CRPv with early left ventricular (LV) dysfunction after STEMI is unknown. The aim of this study was to investigate the relationship between CRPv and early LV dysfunction, either before or at hospital discharge, in patients with first STEMI. This analysis evaluated 432 STEMI patients that were included in the prospective MARINA-STEMI (Magnetic Resonance Imaging In Acute ST-elevation Myocardial Infarction. ClinicalTrials.gov Identifier: NCT04113356) cohort study. The difference of CRP 24 ± 8 h and CRP at hospital admission divided by the time (in h) that elapsed during the two examinations was defined as CRPv. Cardiac magnetic resonance (CMR) imaging was conducted at a median of 3 (IQR 2–4) days after primary percutaneous coronary intervention (PCI) for the determination of LV function and myocardial infarct characteristics. The association of CRPv with the CMR-derived LV ejection fraction (LVEF) was investigated. The median CRPv was 0.42 (IQR 0.21–0.76) mg/l/h and was correlated with LVEF ($r_S = -0.397$, $p < 0.001$). In multivariable linear as well as binary logistic regression analysis (adjustment for biomarkers and clinical and angiographical parameters), CRPv was independently associated with LVEF (β: 0.161, $p = 0.004$) and LVEF ≤ 40% (OR: 1.71, 95% CI: 1.19–2.45; $p = 0.004$), respectively. The combined predictive value of peak cardiac troponin T (cTnT) and CRPv for LVEF ≤ 40% (AUC: 0.81, 95% CI 0.77–0.85, $p < 0.001$) was higher than it was for peak cTnT alone (AUC difference: 0.04, $p = 0.009$). CRPv was independently associated with early LV dysfunction, as measured by the CMR-determined LVEF, revealing an additive predictive value over cTnT after acute STEMI treated with primary PCI.

Keywords: ST-elevation myocardial infarction; C-reactive protein; left ventricular function; cardiac magnetic resonance imaging

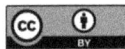

1. Introduction

Despite significant progress in the management of ST-elevation myocardial infarction (STEMI), left ventricular (LV) systolic dysfunction is the most common consequence after STEMI and has significant implications on short- and long-term prognosis [1–3]. Early knowledge of the individual risk of reduced ejection fraction post-STEMI is therefore desirable [4].

Elevated peak C-reactive protein (CRP) levels are associated with reduced LV ejection fraction (LVEF) [5], more severe myocardial tissue injury [6–8], and worse outcome in the setting of acute myocardial infarction [9–11]. However, peak CRP values are reached 2–3 days after acute STEMI, decelerating early risk stratification [6,12]. An association between CRP level dynamics and adverse cardiovascular events and death after acute coronary syndromes has been suggested [13]. According to Świątkiewicz et al., changes in CRP concentrations during STEMI might serve as a risk marker for post-infarct LV systolic dysfunction and heart failure [14–16], even years after the index event, as well as LV remodeling [17], underlining the clinical usefulness of CRP dynamics in this patient setting. In the CAMI-1 study, the CRP gradient was suggested to correlate with a greater extent of myocardial infarct size (IS) and reduced LVEF [18].

CRP velocity (CRPv), which displays CRP level changes over time, has been suggested as a very early and more sensitive parameter for more serious outcomes following STEMI [19–22]. However, the association of CRPv with LV systolic dysfunction has not been specifically investigated so far. The aim of this study was, therefore, to investigate the relationship between CRPv and LVEF, assessed by cardiac magnetic resonance (CMR) imaging, in patients with acute STEMI treated with primary percutaneous coronary intervention (PCI). We hypothesized that CRPv could predict LV dysfunction with a comparable accuracy to peak CRP and peak cardiac troponin T (cTnT) as reference standard biomarkers in this setting.

2. Methods

2.1. Study Design, Patient Population and Endpoint Definition

This study is based on the "Magnetic Resonance Imaging In Acute ST-Elevation Myocardial Infarction (MARINA-STEMI)" trial (ClinicalTrials.gov Identifier: NCT04113356), a prospective observational study recruiting acute STEMI patients, that were treated with primary PCI, at the coronary care unit of the Medical University of Innsbruck. The following inclusion criteria were applied for the present analysis: first STEMI according to the European Society of Cardiology/American College of Cardiology committee criteria [23], revascularization by primary PCI within 12 h after the onset of ischemic signs or symptoms, and Killip class <3 at time of CMR imaging. The exclusion criteria were as follows: inability or unwillingness to sign written informed consent, age < 18 years, any history of a previous myocardial infarction or coronary intervention, high-sensitivity (hs) CRP > 15 mg/L at the time of hospital admission, fever (temperature > 38 °C) or having experienced an acute infection with fever within 14 days prior to study inclusion, chronic inflammatory disease, an estimated glomerular filtration rate < 30 mL/min per 1.73 m^2, and any other contraindication to CMR examination (pacemaker, severe claustrophobia, orbital foreign body, cerebral aneurysm clip, or known or suggested contrast agent allergy to gadolinium) [19].

For the determination of hs-cTnT and hs-CRP, peripheral venous blood samples were performed and analyzed as described previously [24]. In brief, concentrations of CRP were measured on the cobas® 8000 modular analyzer (Roche Diagnostics®), and cTnT measurements were conducted by applying a validated enzyme immunoassay (hs-cTnT; E170, Roche Diagnostics®). CRP and cTnT levels were assessed at hospital admission, 6 ± 2 h, 12 ± 4 h, 24 ± 8 h, and then daily until day 4 after PCI or discharge [25]. The difference between CRP 24 ± 8 h and CRP at hospital admission, divided by the time (in h) that elapsed during the two examinations, was defined as CRPv [19,21].

The primary objective of the current study was the association between CRPv and LVEF as determined by CMR imaging. The secondary objective was to assess the potential additive value of CRPv over cTnT for the prediction of LV dysfunction. The value of LVEF categorization ≤40% to define LV dysfunction is derived from the latest guidelines [26] and is based on previous analyses investigating the prognostic impact of reduced LVEF at any time after STEMI [27].

Prior to study inclusion, all participants gave written informed consent. The study was designed and conducted in accordance with the Declaration of Helsinki and received approval by the research ethics committee of the Medical University of Innsbruck.

2.2. Cardiac Magnetic Resonance Imaging

CMR examinations were performed in the supine position on a 1.5 Tesla clinical MR scanner (MAGNETOM Avanto fit; Siemens Healthineers AG, Erlangen, Germany) within the first week after treatment with primary PCI. The detailed standardized imaging protocol of our research group has been published previously [28]. High-resolution cine images on the long- and short axis covering the LV (10–12 slices) were acquired using a balanced steady state free precession (bSSFP) sequence with retrospective electrocardiographic (ECG) gating [29].

Standard software (Circle Cardiovascular Imaging, Calgary, AB, Canada) was used for post-processing analyses with the semi-automatic detection of LV endo- and epicardial borders [30]. Papillary muscles were excluded from the LV myocardial mass (LVMM) and were included in the LV volume.

An ECG-triggered, phase-sensitive inversion recovery sequence was used to obtain late gadolinium enhancement (LGE) images 15–20 min after the application of 0.2 mmol/kg of Gd-DO3A-butriol (Gadovist®, Bayer Vital GmbH, Leverkusen, Germany), with short-axis slices covering the entire LV [29]. A picture archiving and communication system (PACS) workstation (IMPAX®, Agfa HealthCare, Bonn, Germany) was used for IS quantification, whereas "hyperenhancement" was defined as +5 standard deviations above the signal intensity of remote LV myocardium [31,32]. IS was depicted as the percentage of total LVMM. Microvascular obstruction (MVO) was defined as a persisting area of "hypoenhancement" within the hyperenhanced territory and was also reported as a percentage of LVMM [31]. MVO regions were included in the aggregate IS.

Experienced observers who were blinded to clinical and angiographic data analyzed all of the CMR images.

2.3. Statistical Analyses

SPSS Statistics 27.0.1 (IBM, Armonk, NY, USA) and MedCalc v19.0.7 (Ostend, Belgium) were used for the statistical analyses. Continuous data are depicted as median with interquartile range (IQR), and categorical variables are expressed as numbers with corresponding percentages. The differences in the continuous and categorical variables between two groups were assessed by the Mann–Whitney U-test and Chi-square test, respectively. Correlations between continuous variables were tested with Spearman's rank test. For multivariable testing, linear and binary logistic regression analyses were used to reveal the independent associated markers of LVEF and LVEF $\leq$ 40%, respectively. Parameters indicating significant association ($p < 0.05$) with LVEF and LVEF $\leq$ 40%, respectively, in univariable analysis were inserted into the multivariable model. There were no missing values. Z-scores were calculated to present odds ratios (OR) per 1 standard deviation increase. Receiver operating characteristic (ROC) curve analysis was performed to depict the area under the curve (AUC) for the prediction of LVEF $\leq$ 40%. Comparisons of the ROC curves were conducted according to DeLong et al. [33]. AUC values were classified as negligible ($\leq$0.55), small (0.56–0.63), moderate (0.64–0.70), and strong ($\geq$0.71), following Rice and Harris [34]. For all of the statistical calculations, a two-tailed p-value of <0.05 was defined as significant.

3. Results

3.1. Baseline Patient Characteristics

A total of 432 STEMI patients were included in this analysis. Baseline characteristics of the overall cohort ($n = 432$) as well as separately for patients with LVEF > 40% ($n = 335$, 78%) and LVEF $\leq$ 40% ($n = 97$, 22%) at CMR are depicted in Table 1. The median age of the overall cohort was 57 (IQR 51–65) years. LVEF $\leq$ 40% (22% of patients) was associated with advanced age ($p = 0.010$) and smoking ($p = 0.002$). Total ischemia time was 178 (IQR 120–262) min and did not differ between patients with LVEF $\leq$ 40% and >40% ($p = 0.407$). Patients with LVEF $\leq$ 40% had anterior infarcts more often ($p < 0.001$) as well as lower TIMI flows pre ($p = 0.018$) and post-PCI ($p = 0.006$). No patient had symptomatic heart failure before STEMI. Patients with LVEF $\leq$ 40% had Killip class II more often ($p < 0.001$).

Table 1. Baseline patient characteristics.

	Total Population ($n = 432$)	LVEF > 40% ($n = 335, 78\%$)	LVEF $\leq$ 40% ($n = 97, 22\%$)	p-Value
Age, years	57 [51–65]	56 [50–64]	58 [53–69]	0.010
Female, n (%)	81 (19)	68 (20)	13 (13)	0.125
Body mass index, kg/m^2	26.1 [24.4–28.7]	26.0 [24.4–28.7]	26.2 [24.7–28.7]	0.622
Current smoker, n (%)	247 (57)	205 (61)	42 (43)	0.002
Hyperlipidemia, n (%)	230 (53)	176 (53)	54 (56)	0.586
Diabetes mellitus, n (%)	35 (8)	25 (8)	10 (10)	0.366
Family history, n (%)	135 (31)	112 (33)	23 (24)	0.160
Hypertension, n (%)	191 (44)	148 (44)	43 (44)	0.979
Systolic blood pressure, mmHg	137 [117–154]	136 [117–154]	137 [118–152]	0.827
Diastolic blood pressure, mmHg	82 [72–95]	80 [72–94]	85 [76–100]	0.039
Symptomatic heart failure before STEMI, n (%)	0 (0)	0 (0)	0 (0)	-
Killip class, n (%)				<0.001
I	296 (69)	247 (74)	49 (50)	
II	136 (32)	88 (26)	48 (50)	
Total ischemia time, min	178 [120–262]	171 [120–260]	188 [129–267]	0.407
Culprit lesion, n (%)				<0.001
RCA	183 (42)	165 (49)	18 (19)	
LAD	189 (44)	124 (37)	65 (67)	
LCX	57 (13)	45 (13)	12 (12)	
RI	3 (1)	1 (1)	2 (2)	
Anterior infarction, n (%)	190 (44)	126 (38)	64 (66)	<0.001
Number of affected vessels, n (%)				0.656
1	260 (60)	201 (60)	59 (61)	
2	119 (28)	95 (28)	24 (25)	
3	53 (12)	39 (12)	14 (14)	
TIMI flow pre-PCI, n (%)				0.018
0	273 (63)	200 (60)	73 (75)	
1	55 (13)	43 (13)	12 (13)	
2	75 (17)	67 (20)	8 (8)	
3	29 (7)	25 (7)	4 (4)	
TIMI flow post-PCI, n (%)				0.006
0	4 (1)	2 (1)	2 (2)	
1	6 (1)	3 (1)	3 (3)	
2	34 (8)	20 (6)	14 (14)	
3	388 (90)	310 (92)	78 (81)	
CRP, mg/L				
Admission	2.1 [1.0–4.2]	2.0 [1.0–4.2]	2.3 [1.0–4.7]	0.383
24 h	12.4 [6.9–20.1]	11.0 [6.0–17.1]	20.9 [10.9–45.7]	<0.001
Peak	22.5 [11.7–45.5]	19.0 [10.3–34.4]	54.6 [25.9–94.7]	<0.001
Admission to 24 h CRP, h	21 [19–25]	21 [19–25]	21 [19–25]	0.640
Admission to peak CRP, h	46 [35–56]	45 [31–55]	47 [42–58]	0.028
CRPv (admission to 24 h), mg/L/h	0.42 [0.21–0.76]	0.34 [0.16–0.61]	0.81 [0.47–1.78]	<0.001
cTnT, ng/L				
Peak	4646 [2187–8430]	3902 [1718–6676]	9065 [5014–14877]	<0.001
Admission to peak cTnT, h	11 [7–16]	11 [7–16]	9 [6–13]	0.014

CRP = C-reactive protein, CRPv = C-reactive protein velocity, cTnT = cardiac troponin T, LAD = left anterior descending artery, LCX = left circumflex artery, LVEF = left ventricular ejection fraction, PCI = percutaneous coronary intervention, RCA = right coronary artery, RI = ramus intermedius, TIMI = thrombolysis in myocardial infarction.

The values for the median admission CRP, 24 h, and peak CRP were as follows: 2.1 (IQR 1.0–4.2), 12.4 (IQR 6.9–20.1), and 22.5 (IQR 11.7–45.5) mg/L, respectively. The median CRPv was 0.42 (IQR 0.21–0.76) mg/L/h and was significantly higher in patients with LVEF $\leq$ 40% ($p < 0.001$) (Figure 1).

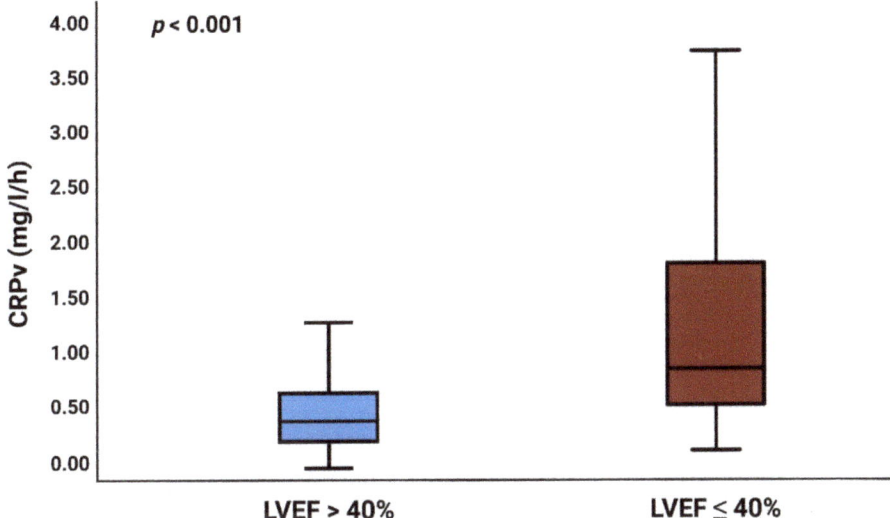

Figure 1. Boxplot showing the relation between CRPv and LVEF. CRPv = C-reactive protein velocity, LVEF = left ventricular ejection fraction.

The median time from PCI to CMR was 3 (IQR 2–4) days. Table 2 provides the CMR parameters of the overall cohort and according to the dichotomized LVEF at 40%.

Table 2. CMR imaging results.

	Total Population ($n = 432$)	LVEF > 40% ($n = 335, 78\%$)	LVEF $\leq$ 40% ($n = 97, 22\%$)	p-Value
LVEDV, mL	167 [137–189]	162 [134–187]	182 [154–204]	<0.001
LVESV, mL	83 [64–94]	75 [60–92]	118 [99–131]	<0.001
LVEF, %	49 [42–55]	-	-	-
LVSV, mL	79 [65–94]	84 [70–97]	60 [50–75]	<0.001
CO, L/min	5.3 [4.4–6.2]	5.5 [4.7–6.3]	4.6 [3.8–5.7]	<0.001
IS, % of LVMM	14.5 [7.5–24.3]	13.0 [6.2–20.6]	26.1 [16.0–34.2]	<0.001
MVO, n (%)	241 (56)	160 (48)	81 (84)	<0.001
MVO, % of LVMM	0.4 [0.0–2.5]	0.0 [0.0–1.5]	2.5 [0.6–6.4]	<0.001

CMR = cardiac magnetic resonance, CO = cardiac output, IS = infarct size, LVEDV = left ventricular end-diastolic volume, LVESV = left ventricular end-systolic volume, LVEF = left ventricular ejection fraction, LVMM = left ventricular myocardial mass, LVSV = left ventricular stroke volume, MVO = microvascular obstruction.

3.2. CRPv as a Marker of LV Dysfunction

CRPv was correlated with LVEF ($r_S = -0.397$, $p < 0.001$). In multiple linear regression analysis, CRPv (β: −0.161, $p = 0.004$), peak cTnT (β: −0.343, $p < 0.001$), TIMI flow pre-PCI (β: 0.085, $p = 0.045$), TIMI flow post-PCI (β: 0.105, $p = 0.010$), and current smoking (β: 0.104, $p = 0.015$) were significantly related to LVEF (Table 3). After binary logistic regression analysis, CRPv (OR 1.71, 95% confidence interval (CI) 1.19–2.45; $p = 0.004$) and peak cTnT (OR 2.09, 95% CI 1.54–2.85; $p < 0.001$) remained independently associated with LVEF $\leq$ 40% (Table 4). In ROC analysis, 24 h CRP (AUC 0.73, 95% CI 0.69–0.77; $p < 0.001$), CRPv (AUC 0.77, 95% CI 0.72–0.81; $p < 0.001$), peak CRP (AUC 0.77, 95% CI 0.73–0.81; $p < 0.001$), and peak cTnT (AUC 0.77, 95% CI 0.73–0.81; $p < 0.001$) emerged as strong predictors of LVEF $\leq$ 40%. The best cut-off value of CRPv in predicting LVEF $\leq$ 40% was >0.59 mg/l/h, with a sensitivity of 70% and a specificity of 75%. According to C-statistics, the AUCs of CRPv and peak CRP (AUC difference: <0.01, p = 0.807) and CRPv and peak cTnT (AUC difference: <0.01, p = 0.784) did not differ. The combination of peak cTnT and CRPv (AUC: 0.81, 95% CI 0.77–0.85, p < 0.001) resulted in a higher AUC than peak cTnT alone for the prediction of LVEF ≤ 40% (AUC difference: 0.04, p = 0.009) (Table 5). The statistical significance of the calibration performance according to the Hosmer–Lemeshow test of the combination of CRPv and TnT was p = 0.063. Internal validity was assessed in 1000 bootstrap samples to estimate the optimism-corrected confidence intervals of the AUC of the combination of CRPv and TnT (BCa 95% CI 0.76–0.86, p < 0.001).

Table 3. Linear regression analysis for the prediction of LVEF.

	Univariable		Multivariable	
	β	p-Value	β	p-Value
CRPv	−0.397	<0.001	−0.161	0.004
Peak CRP	−0.378	<0.001	−0.098	0.082
Peak cTnT	−0.498	<0.001	−0.343	<0.001
Anterior infarction	−0.222	<0.001	−0.047	0.253
TIMI flow pre-PCI	0.264	<0.001	0.085	0.045
TIMI flow post-PCI	0.204	<0.001	0.105	0.010
Current smoker	0.173	<0.001	0.104	0.015
Age	−0.133	0.006	0.011	0.806
Diastolic blood pressure	0.000	0.999	-	-
Killip class	−0.210	<0.001	−0.053	0.197

CRP = C-reactive protein, CRPv = C-reactive protein velocity, cTnT = cardiac troponin T, LVEF = left ventricular ejection fraction, PCI = percutaneous coronary intervention. TIMI = thrombolysis in myocardial infarction.

Table 4. Binary logistic regression analysis for the prediction of LVEF ≤ 40%.

	Univariable		Multivariable	
	OR (95% CI)	p-Value	OR (95% CI)	p-Value
CRPv	2.69 (2.01–3.60)	<0.001	1.71 (1.19–2.45)	0.004
Peak CRP	2.55 (1.92–3.39)	<0.001	1.28 (0.92–1.79)	0.146
Peak cTnT	2.82 (2.15–3.71)	<0.001	2.09 (1.54–2.85)	<0.001
Anterior infarction	1.78 (1.41–2.26)	<0.001	1.28 (0.97–1.71)	0.079
TIMI flow pre-PCI	0.67 (0.51–0.88)	0.003	1.04 (0.75–1.44)	0.828
TIMI flow post-PCI	0.73 (0.60–0.89)	0.002	0.83 (0.65–1.05)	0.112
Current smoker	0.70 (0.56–0.88)	0.002	0.76 (0.56–1.03)	0.079
Age	1.38 (1.09–1.72)	0.006	1.03 (0.75–1.37)	0.914
Diastolic blood pressure	1.27 (1.02–1.59)	0.037	1.18 (0.89–1.55)	0.258
Killip class	2.75 (1.72–4.38)	<0.001	1.54 (0.87–2.76)	0.142

CI = confidence interval, CRP = C-reactive protein, CRPv = C-reactive protein velocity, cTnT = cardiac troponin T, LVEF = left ventricular ejection fraction, OR = odds ratio, PCI = percutaneous coronary intervention. TIMI = thrombolysis in myocardial infarction. OR are presented per 1 standard deviation increase.

Table 5. C-statistics for the prediction of LVEF ≤ 40%.

Variables	AUC	95% CI	p-Value	AUC Increment	ROC Comparison
Admission CRP	0.53	0.48–0.58	0.383	-	-
24 h CRP	0.73	0.69–0.77	<0.001	0.20	<0.001
CRPv	0.77	0.72–0.81	<0.001	0.04	<0.001
Peak CRP	0.77	0.73–0.81	<0.001	<0.01	0.807
Peak cTnT	0.77	0.73–0.81	<0.001	<0.01	0.905
CRPv and peak cTnT	0.81	0.77–0.85	<0.001	0.04	0.009

AUC = area under the curve, CI = confidence interval, CRP = C-reactive protein, cTnT = cardiac troponin T, LVEF = left ventricular ejection fraction, ROC = receiver operating characteristic.

4. Discussion

The present study investigated the association of CRPv with LV dysfunction as assessed by CMR in patients with acute STEMI treated with primary PCI for the first time.

The major findings can be summarized as follows: (a) Patients with elevated CRPv levels had significantly lower LVEF. (b) In the first week following acute STEMI, the association of CRPv and LV dysfunction remained significant after adjustment for clinical (peak CRP, peak cTnT, smoking, age, Killip class) and angiographical parameters (anterior infarct localization, TIMI flow pre- and post-PCI). (c) The predictive value of CRPv for LVEF $\leq 40\%$ was strong and additive to peak cTnT. Taken together, these data indicate that CRPv represents a sensitive risk stratification tool in daily clinical practice, that is available in the very early phase after STEMI. Moreover, further studies could explore whether patients with increased CRP levels could benefit from individualized therapeutic strategies targeting the post-STEMI inflammatory response.

Among several inflammatory markers in the setting of myocardial infarction, CRP represents the most intensively explored marker. As an acute phase protein, CRP is released by hepatocytes after the stimulation of cytokines, primarily interleukin-6, about 6 h after the beginning of ischemic injury and peaks at day 2–3 thereafter [6,12]. Interleukin-6 is considered to increase the risk of adverse events after an acute coronary syndrome [35]. Furthermore, existing evidence shows that ischemic cell damage by CRP is complement dependent [36]. Increased CRP levels are associated with a greater extent of myocardial tissue damage [6–8,18], more severe LV dysfunction [18,37], and the occurrence of adverse events [9–11] after myocardial infarction. Furthermore, persisting inflammatory response in the chronic phase after STEMI can contribute to adverse LV remodeling [38]. CRP might therefore serve as an early biomarker for risk stratification after infarction.

Changes in CRP concentrations during myocardial infarction are considered to play a crucial role regarding adverse cardiovascular events, including death [13] and LV dysfunction, even years later [14]. In a study by Świątkiewicz et al. investigating 204 patients with first STEMI, elevated serial CRP during STEMI was associated with an increased risk of LV systolic dysfunction and heart failure [16]. Furthermore, elevated CRP values are also suggested to predict LV remodeling in this patient population [17].

Dynamics in inflammatory processes during myocardial infarction, as measured by CRPv, have recently been shown to predict microvascular pathology [19], which is a major prognostic determinant after STEMI [39]. In line with this, another study indicated that CRPv might be associated with short-term mortality after STEMI [21]. Moreover, CRPv is not only associated with a risk for adverse outcomes after STEMI, but is also related to the onset of new atrial fibrillation [20]. Atrial fibrillation is known to predict adverse outcomes after STEMI [40]. Furthermore, Zahler et al. revealed an association between CRPv and acute kidney injury after STEMI [22]. In the present study, we could corroborate and expand previous findings by showing that CRPv is strongly and independently associated with LV dysfunction after acute STEMI. In particular, this study may have clinical and research implications: firstly, CRPv emerged as an early and sensitive parameter for the prediction of LV dysfunction, as measured by CMR-assessed LVEF, improving individual risk assessment in this patient population at a very early stage. Secondly, as elevated CRPv levels are indicative for reduced LVEF in this study, CRPv may help to identify patients who might benefit from an anti-inflammatory and more extensive cardio protective treatment [41]. This hypothesis needs to be addressed in further studies.

Another important research question is whether CRP is only an associate or a mechanistic (causal) driver of LV dysfunction after STEMI. Indeed, the modulation of inflammatory processes have recently moved more and more into focus in the treatment of STEMI. The recently published CAMI-1 study [18] revealed that the CRP gradient was correlated with a greater extent of myocardial IS and reduced LVEF. By lowering CRP concentrations with CRP apheresis, the authors concluded that the correlation between CRP and myocardial IS and LV dysfunction was no longer detectable. The promising role of selective CRP apheresis in this setting needs further evaluation. The currently ongoing, prospective, randomized controlled "CRP Apheresis in STEMI" trial (ClinicalTrials.gov Identifier: NCT04939805) is investigating the effect of selective CRP apheresis on IS after acute STEMI and will provide important insights [42]. Moreover, the ASSAIL-MI trial [43] revealed that the intraprocedural administration of the interleukin-6 inhibitor Tocilizumab led to significant CRP reduction and consequently to an increased myocardial salvage, as assessed by CMR. Nevertheless, there was no difference in LVEF and IS between the experimental and control group. In experimental models, NLRP3 (NOD-like receptor family, pyrin domain-containing 3) inflammasome-targeted strategies might be beneficial in acute myocardial infarction [44]. In a mouse model of ischemia-reperfusion injury, the inhibition of NLRP3 inflammasomes has been shown to preserve myocardial function [45]. Another anti-inflammatory therapeutic strategy might be interleukin-1 blockade with anakinra, which has been suggested to potentially prevent heart failure after acute myocardial infarction [46]. Canakinumab, an interleukin-1b inhibitor, has been considered to have a dose-dependent reduction in the occurrence of heart failure in patients with prior myocardial infarction and elevated CRP [47]. However, research in this field is warranted to point out possible future directives in anti-inflammatory therapies after myocardial infarction.

To summarize, CRPv could help in the characterization of the dynamic inflammatory mechanism in the setting of acute STEMI as a time-dependent parameter and has important implications on myocardial infarct characteristics and outcome [19], as well as on remnant LV function before or at hospital discharge upon STEMI.

Limitations

In this study, only stable STEMI patients with Killip class < 3 and a delay < 12 h were included [19]. The majority of STEMI patients present with Killip class < 3 [48]. However, the association of CRPv and LVEF might thus not be applicable to unstable patients, to late presenters, and to NSTEMI. Moreover, the results of this analysis might not be applicable to patients with symptomatic heart failure before STEMI. The TIMI myocardial perfusion grade was not systematically assessed in this cohort, although it might be a better discriminator than TIMI flow post PCI for poor prognosis after STEMI [49,50]. Furthermore, our scientific explanations are not transmissive to patients with an increased admission CRP value (above 15 mg/L), which are, however, a very small minority of patients (<4%) [19]. Finally, this study investigated the impact of CRPv on early LV dysfunction; thus, the results might not be transmissive to patients with LV dysfunction occurring in the chronic phase after STEMI. Further validation and research is needed to describe the exact role and significance of CRPv in this setting.

5. Conclusions

CRPv is independently associated with LV dysfunction, as determined by CMR, before or at hospital discharge in patients with acute STEMI treated with primary PCI. CRPv might help to identify patients who are at an increased risk for LV dysfunction at a very early stage after STEMI.

Author Contributions: M.H.: study conception and design, analysis and interpretation of data, drafting of the manuscript, final approval of the manuscript; C.T.: analysis and interpretation of data, critical revision of the manuscript for important intellectual content, final approval of the manuscript; M.R.: analysis and interpretation of data, critical revision of the manuscript for important intellectual content, final approval of the manuscript; I.L.: analysis and interpretation of data, critical revision of the manuscript for important intellectual content, final approval of the manuscript; P.F.: analysis and interpretation of data, critical revision of the manuscript for important intellectual content, final approval of the manuscript; P.L.: analysis and interpretation of data, critical revision of the manuscript for important intellectual content, final approval of the manuscript; A.M.: analysis and interpretation of data, critical revision of the manuscript for important intellectual content, final approval of the manuscript; B.H.: analysis and interpretation of data, critical revision of the manuscript for important intellectual content, final approval of the manuscript; C.B.: analysis and interpretation of data, critical revision of the manuscript for important intellectual content, final approval of the manuscript; G.K.: analysis and interpretation of data, critical revision of the manuscript for important intellectual content, final approval of the manuscript; A.B.: analysis and interpretation of data, critical revision of the manuscript for important intellectual content, final approval of the manuscript. B.M.

study conception and design, analysis and interpretation of data, drafting of the manuscript, final approval of the manuscript; S.J.R. (corresponding author): study conception and design, analysis and interpretation of data, drafting of the manuscript, final approval of the manuscript. All authors have read and agreed to the published version of the manuscript.

Funding: The "Austrian Society of Cardiology", "Tiroler Wissenschaftsförderung" and the "Austrian Science Fund" (FWF grant KLI 772-B).

Institutional Review Board Statement: The study was conducted according to the guidelines of the Declaration of Helsinki, and approved by the Institutional Review Board (Ethics Committee) of the Medical University of Innsbruck (protocol code: AN3775, date of approval: 4 November 2009).

Informed Consent Statement: Informed consent was obtained from all subjects involved in the study.

Acknowledgments: The study was supported by grants from the "Austrian Society of Cardiology", "Tiroler Wissenschaftsförderung", and the "Austrian Science Fund" (FWF grant KLI 772-B).

Conflicts of Interest: All authors have declared no conflict of interest.

References

1. Desta, L.; Jernberg, T.; Lofman, I.; Hofman-Bang, C.; Hagerman, I.; Spaak, J.; Persson, H. Incidence, temporal trends, and prognostic impact of heart failure complicating acute myocardial infarction. The SWEDEHEART Registry (Swedish Web-System for Enhancement and Development of Evidence-Based Care in Heart Disease Evaluated According to Recommended Therapies): A study of 199,851 patients admitted with index acute myocardial infarctions, 1996 to 2008. *JACC Heart Fail.* **2015**, *3*, 234–242. [PubMed]
2. Sutton, N.R.; Li, S.; Thomas, L.; Wang, T.Y.; de Lemos, J.A.; Enriquez, J.R.; Shah, R.U.; Fonarow, G.C. The association of left ventricular ejection fraction with clinical outcomes after myocardial infarction: Findings from the Acute Coronary Treatment and Intervention Outcomes Network (ACTION) Registry-Get With the Guidelines (GWTG) Medicare-linked database. *Am. Heart J.* **2016**, *178*, 65–73. [CrossRef] [PubMed]
3. Ng, V.G.; Lansky, A.J.; Meller, S.; Witzenbichler, B.; Guagliumi, G.; Peruga, J.Z.; Brodie, B.; Shah, R.; Mehran, R.; Stone, G.W. The prognostic importance of left ventricular function in patients with ST-segment elevation myocardial infarction: The HORIZONS-AMI trial. *Eur. Heart J. Acute Cardiovasc. Care* **2014**, *3*, 67–77. [CrossRef] [PubMed]
4. Ponikowski, P.; Voors, A.A.; Anker, S.D.; Bueno, H.; Cleland, J.G.F.; Coats, A.J.S.; Falk, V.; Gonzalez-Juanatey, J.R.; Harjola, V.P.; Jankowska, E.A.; et al. 2016 ESC Guidelines for the diagnosis and treatment of acute and chronic heart failure: The Task Force for the diagnosis and treatment of acute and chronic heart failure of the European Society of Cardiology (ESC) Developed with the special contribution of the Heart Failure Association (HFA) of the ESC. *Eur. Heart J.* **2016**, *37*, 2129–2200. [PubMed]
5. Stumpf, C.; Sheriff, A.; Zimmermann, S.; Schaefauer, L.; Schlundt, C.; Raaz, D.; Garlichs, C.D.; Achenbach, S. C-reactive protein levels predict systolic heart failure and outcome in patients with first ST-elevation myocardial infarction treated with coronary angioplasty. *Arch. Med. Sci.* **2017**, *13*, 1086–1093. [CrossRef]
6. Reindl, M.; Reinstadler, S.J.; Feistritzer, H.J.; Klug, G.; Tiller, C.; Mair, J.; Mayr, A.; Jaschke, W.; Metzler, B. Relation of inflammatory markers with myocardial and microvascular injury in patients with reperfused ST-elevation myocardial infarction. *Eur. Heart J. Acute Cardiovasc. Care* **2017**, *6*, 640–649. [CrossRef]
7. Mather, A.N.; Fairbairn, T.A.; Artis, N.J.; Greenwood, J.P.; Plein, S. Relationship of cardiac biomarkers and reversible and irreversible myocardial injury following acute myocardial infarction as determined by cardiovascular magnetic resonance. *Int J. Cardiol.* **2013**, *166*, 458–464. [CrossRef]
8. Orn, S.; Manhenke, C.; Ueland, T.; Damas, J.K.; Mollnes, T.E.; Edvardsen, T.; Aukrust, P.; Dickstein, K. C-reactive protein, infarct size, microvascular obstruction, and left-ventricular remodelling following acute myocardial infarction. *Eur. Heart J.* **2009**, *30*, 1180–1186. [CrossRef]
9. Yip, H.K.; Hang, C.L.; Fang, C.Y.; Hsieh, Y.K.; Yang, C.H.; Hung, W.C.; Wu, C.J. Level of high-sensitivity C-reactive protein is predictive of 30-day outcomes in patients with acute myocardial infarction undergoing primary coronary intervention. *Chest* **2005**, *127*, 803–808. [CrossRef]
10. Theroux, P.; Armstrong, P.W.; Mahaffey, K.W.; Hochman, J.S.; Malloy, K.J.; Rollins, S.; Nicolau, J.C.; Lavoie, J.; Luong, T.M.; Burchenal, J.; et al. Prognostic significance of blood markers of inflammation in patients with ST-segment elevation myocardial infarction undergoing primary angioplasty and effects of pexelizumab, a C5 inhibitor: A substudy of the COMMA trial. *Eur. Heart J.* **2005**, *26*, 1964–1970. [CrossRef]
11. Ortolani, P.; Marzocchi, A.; Marrozzini, C.; Palmerini, T.; Saia, F.; Taglieri, N.; Baldazzi, F.; Silenzi, S.; Bacchi-Reggiani, M.L.; Guastaroba, P.; et al. Predictive value of high sensitivity C-reactive protein in patients with ST-elevation myocardial infarction treated with percutaneous coronary intervention. *Eur. Heart J.* **2008**, *29*, 1241–1249. [CrossRef]
12. Kushner, I.; Broder, M.L.; Karp, D. Control of the acute phase response. Serum C-reactive protein kinetics after acute myocardial infarction. *J. Clin. Investig.* **1978**, *61*, 235–242. [CrossRef]

13. Mani, P.; Puri, R.; Schwartz, G.G.; Nissen, S.E.; Shao, M.; Kastelein, J.J.P.; Menon, V.; Lincoff, A.M.; Nicholls, S.J. Association of Initial and Serial C-Reactive Protein Levels With Adverse Cardiovascular Events and Death After Acute Coronary Syndrome: A Secondary Analysis of the VISTA-16 Trial. *JAMA Cardiol.* **2019**, *4*, 314–320. [CrossRef]
14. Swiatkiewicz, I.; Magielski, P.; Kubica, J. C-Reactive Protein as a Risk Marker for Post-Infarct Heart Failure over a Multi-Year Period. *Int. J. Mol. Sci.* **2021**, *22*, 3169. [CrossRef]
15. Swiatkiewicz, I.; Taub, P.R. The usefulness of C-reactive protein for the prediction of post-infarct left ventricular systolic dysfunction and heart failure. *Kardiol. Pol.* **2018**, *76*, 821–829. [CrossRef]
16. Swiatkiewicz, I.; Magielski, P.; Kubica, J.; Zadourian, A.; DeMaria, A.N.; Taub, P.R. Enhanced Inflammation is a Marker for Risk of Post-Infarct Ventricular Dysfunction and Heart Failure. *Int. J. Mol. Sci.* **2020**, *21*, 807. [CrossRef]
17. Swiatkiewicz, I.; Kozinski, M.; Magielski, P.; Fabiszak, T.; Sukiennik, A.; Navarese, E.P.; Odrowaz-Sypniewska, G.; Kubica, J. Value of C-reactive protein in predicting left ventricular remodelling in patients with a first ST-segment elevation myocardial infarction. *Mediat. Inflamm.* **2012**, *2012*, 250867. [CrossRef]
18. Ries, W.; Torzewski, J.; Heigl, F.; Pfluecke, C.; Kelle, S.; Darius, H.; Ince, H.; Mitzner, S.; Nordbeck, P.; Butter, C.; et al. C-Reactive Protein Apheresis as Anti-inflammatory Therapy in Acute Myocardial Infarction: Results of the CAMI-1 Study. *Front. Cardiovasc. Med.* **2021**, *8*, 591714. [CrossRef]
19. Holzknecht, M.; Tiller, C.; Reindl, M.; Lechner, I.; Troger, F.; Hosp, M.; Mayr, A.; Brenner, C.; Klug, G.; Bauer, A.; et al. C-reactive protein velocity predicts microvascular pathology after acute ST-elevation myocardial infarction. *Int. J. Cardiol.* **2021**. [CrossRef]
20. Zahler, D.; Merdler, I.; Rozenfeld, K.L.; Shenberg, G.; Milwidsky, A.; Berliner, S.; Banai, S.; Arbel, Y.; Shacham, Y. C-Reactive Protein Velocity and the Risk of New Onset Atrial Fibrillation among ST Elevation Myocardial Infarction Patients. *Isr. Med. Assoc. J.* **2021**, *23*, 169–173.
21. Milwidsky, A.; Ziv-Baran, T.; Letourneau-Shesaf, S.; Keren, G.; Taieb, P.; Berliner, S.; Shacham, Y. CRP velocity and short-term mortality in ST segment elevation myocardial infarction. *Biomarkers* **2017**, *22*, 383–386. [CrossRef]
22. Zahler, D.; Rozenfeld, K.L.; Stein, M.; Milwidsky, A.; Berliner, S.; Banai, S.; Arbel, Y.; Shacham, Y. C-reactive protein velocity and the risk of acute kidney injury among ST elevation myocardial infarction patients undergoing primary percutaneous intervention. *J. Nephrol.* **2019**, *32*, 437–443. [CrossRef]
23. Thygesen, K.; Alpert, J.S.; Jaffe, A.S.; Chaitman, B.R.; Bax, J.J.; Morrow, D.A.; White, H.D.; Group, E.S.C.S.D. Fourth universal definition of myocardial infarction (2018). *Eur. Heart J.* **2019**, *40*, 237–269. [CrossRef]
24. Reinstadler, S.J.; Feistritzer, H.J.; Klug, G.; Mair, J.; Tu, A.M.; Kofler, M.; Henninger, B.; Franz, W.M.; Metzler, B. High-sensitivity troponin T for prediction of left ventricular function and infarct size one year following ST-elevation myocardial infarction. *Int. J. Cardiol.* **2016**, *202*, 188–193. [CrossRef]
25. Feistritzer, H.J.; Reinstadler, S.J.; Klug, G.; Reindl, M.; Wohrer, S.; Brenner, C.; Mayr, A.; Mair, J.; Metzler, B. Multimarker approach for the prediction of microvascular obstruction after acute ST-segment elevation myocardial infarction: A prospective, observational study. *BMC Cardiovasc. Disord.* **2016**, *16*, 239. [CrossRef]
26. McDonagh, T.A.; Metra, M.; Adamo, M.; Gardner, R.S.; Baumbach, A.; Bohm, M.; Burri, H.; Butler, J.; Celutkiene, J.; Chioncel, O.; et al. 2021 ESC Guidelines for the diagnosis and treatment of acute and chronic heart failure. *Eur. Heart J.* **2021**, *42*, 3599–3726. [CrossRef]
27. Gavara, J.; Marcos-Garces, V.; Lopez-Lereu, M.P.; Monmeneu, J.V.; Rios-Navarro, C.; de Dios, E.; Perez, N.; Merenciano, H.; Gabaldon, A.; Canoves, J.; et al. Magnetic Resonance Assessment of Left Ventricular Ejection Fraction at Any Time Post-Infarction for Prediction of Subsequent Events in a Large Multicenter STEMI Registry. *J. Magn. Reson. Imaging* **2021**. [CrossRef] [PubMed]
28. Reinstadler, S.J.; Klug, G.; Feistritzer, H.J.; Mayr, A.; Harrasser, B.; Mair, J.; Bader, K.; Streil, K.; Hammerer-Lercher, A.; Esterhammer, R.; et al. Association of copeptin with myocardial infarct size and myocardial function after ST segment elevation myocardial infarction. *Heart* **2013**, *99*, 1525–1529. [CrossRef] [PubMed]
29. Holzknecht, M.; Reindl, M.; Tiller, C.; Reinstadler, S.J.; Lechner, I.; Pamminger, M.; Schwaiger, J.P.; Klug, G.; Bauer, A.; Metzler, B.; et al. Global longitudinal strain improves risk assessment after ST-segment elevation myocardial infarction: A comparative prognostic evaluation of left ventricular functional parameters. *Clin. Res. Cardiol.* **2021**, *110*, 1599–1611. [CrossRef] [PubMed]
30. Lechner, I.; Reindl, M.; Tiller, C.; Holzknecht, M.; Troger, F.; Fink, P.; Mayr, A.; Klug, G.; Bauer, A.; Metzler, B.; et al. Impact of COVID-19 pandemic restrictions on ST-segment elevation myocardial infarction: A cardiac MRI study. *Eur. Heart J.* **2021**, ehab621. [CrossRef] [PubMed]
31. Reindl, M.; Reinstadler, S.J.; Feistritzer, H.J.; Theurl, M.; Basic, D.; Eigler, C.; Holzknecht, M.; Mair, J.; Mayr, A.; Klug, G.; et al. Relation of Low-Density Lipoprotein Cholesterol with Microvascular Injury and Clinical Outcome in Revascularized ST-Elevation Myocardial Infarction. *J. Am. Heart Assoc.* **2017**, *6*, e006957. [CrossRef]
32. Bondarenko, O.; Beek, A.M.; Hofman, M.B.; Kuhl, H.P.; Twisk, J.W.; van Dockum, W.G.; Visser, C.A.; van Rossum, A.C. Standardizing the definition of hyperenhancement in the quantitative assessment of infarct size and myocardial viability using delayed contrast-enhanced CMR. *J. Cardiovasc. Magn. Reson.* **2005**, *7*, 481–485. [CrossRef]
33. DeLong, E.R.; DeLong, D.M.; Clarke-Pearson, D.L. Comparing the areas under two or more correlated receiver operating characteristic curves: A nonparametric approach. *Biometrics* **1988**, *44*, 837–845. [CrossRef]
34. Rice, M.E.; Harris, G.T. Comparing effect sizes in follow-up studies: ROC Area, Cohen's d, and r. *Law Hum. Behav.* **2005**, *29*, 615–620. [CrossRef]

35. Fanola, C.L.; Morrow, D.A.; Cannon, C.P.; Jarolim, P.; Lukas, M.A.; Bode, C.; Hochman, J.S.; Goodrich, E.L.; Braunwald, E.; O'Donoghue, M.L. Interleukin-6 and the Risk of Adverse Outcomes in Patients After an Acute Coronary Syndrome: Observations From the SOLID-TIMI 52 (Stabilization of Plaque Using Darapladib-Thrombolysis in Myocardial Infarction 52) Trial. *J. Am. Heart Assoc.* **2017**, *6*, e005637. [CrossRef]
36. Sheriff, A.; Kayser, S.; Brunner, P.; Vogt, B. C-Reactive Protein Triggers Cell Death in Ischemic Cells. *Front. Immunol.* **2021**, *12*, 630430. [CrossRef]
37. Vanhaverbeke, M.; Veltman, D.; Pattyn, N.; De Crem, N.; Gillijns, H.; Cornelissen, V.; Janssens, S.; Sinnaeve, P.R. C-reactive protein during and after myocardial infarction in relation to cardiac injury and left ventricular function at follow-up. *Clin. Cardiol.* **2018**, *41*, 1201–1206. [CrossRef]
38. Tiller, C.; Reindl, M.; Holzknecht, M.; Lechner, I.; Simma, F.; Schwaiger, J.; Mayr, A.; Klug, G.; Bauer, A.; Reinstadler, S.J.; et al. High sensitivity C-reactive protein is associated with worse infarct healing after revascularized ST-elevation myocardial infarction. *Int. J. Cardiol.* **2020**, *328*, 191–196. [CrossRef]
39. de Waha, S.; Patel, M.R.; Granger, C.B.; Ohman, E.M.; Maehara, A.; Eitel, I.; Ben-Yehuda, O.; Jenkins, P.; Thiele, H.; Stone, G.W. Relationship between microvascular obstruction and adverse events following primary percutaneous coronary intervention for ST-segment elevation myocardial infarction: An individual patient data pooled analysis from seven randomized trials. *Eur. Heart J.* **2017**, *38*, 3502–3510. [CrossRef]
40. Reinstadler, S.J.; Stiermaier, T.; Eitel, C.; Fuernau, G.; Saad, M.; Poss, J.; de Waha, S.; Mende, M.; Desch, S.; Metzler, B.; et al. Impact of Atrial Fibrillation During ST-Segment-Elevation Myocardial Infarction on Infarct Characteristics and Prognosis. *Circ. Cardiovasc. Imaging* **2018**, *11*, e006955. [CrossRef]
41. Montone, R.A.; La Vecchia, G. Interplay between inflammation and microvascular obstruction in ST-segment elevation myocardial infarction: The importance of velocity. *Int J. Cardiol.* **2021**, *339*, 7–9. [CrossRef]
42. ClinicalTrials.gov. CRP Apheresis in STEMI. Available online: https://clinicaltrials.gov/ct2/show/NCT04939805 (accessed on 27 September 2021).
43. Broch, K.; Anstensrud, A.K.; Woxholt, S.; Sharma, K.; Tollefsen, I.M.; Bendz, B.; Aakhus, S.; Ueland, T.; Amundsen, B.H.; Damas, J.K.; et al. Randomized Trial of Interleukin-6 Receptor Inhibition in Patients with Acute ST-Segment Elevation Myocardial Infarction. *J. Am. Coll. Cardiol.* **2021**, *77*, 1845–1855. [CrossRef]
44. Toldo, S.; Abbate, A. The NLRP3 inflammasome in acute myocardial infarction. *Nat. Rev. Cardiol.* **2018**, *15*, 203–214. [CrossRef]
45. Abbate, A.; Toldo, S.; Marchetti, C.; Kron, J.; Van Tassell, B.W.; Dinarello, C.A. Interleukin-1 and the Inflammasome as Therapeutic Targets in Cardiovascular Disease. *Circ. Res.* **2020**, *126*, 1260–1280. [CrossRef]
46. Abbate, A.; Kontos, M.C.; Grizzard, J.D.; Biondi-Zoccai, G.G.; Van Tassell, B.W.; Robati, R.; Roach, L.M.; Arena, R.A.; Roberts, C.S.; Varma, A.; et al. Interleukin-1 blockade with anakinra to prevent adverse cardiac remodeling after acute myocardial infarction (Virginia Commonwealth University Anakinra Remodeling Trial [VCU-ART] Pilot study). *Am. J. Cardiol.* **2010**, *105*, 1371–1377.e1. [CrossRef]
47. Everett, B.M.; Cornel, J.H.; Lainscak, M.; Anker, S.D.; Abbate, A.; Thuren, T.; Libby, P.; Glynn, R.J.; Ridker, P.M. Anti-Inflammatory Therapy with Canakinumab for the Prevention of Hospitalization for Heart Failure. *Circulation* **2019**, *139*, 1289–1299. [CrossRef]
48. El-Menyar, A.; Zubaid, M.; AlMahmeed, W.; Sulaiman, K.; AlNabti, A.; Singh, R.; Al Suwaidi, J. Killip classification in patients with acute coronary syndrome: Insight from a multicenter registry. *Am. J. Emerg. Med.* **2012**, *30*, 97–103. [CrossRef]
49. Overtchouk, P.; Barthelemy, O.; Hauguel-Moreau, M.; Guedeney, P.; Rouanet, S.; Zeitouni, M.; Silvain, J.; Collet, J.P.; Vicaut, E.; Zeymer, U.; et al. Angiographic predictors of outcome in myocardial infarction patients presenting with cardiogenic shock: A CULPRIT-SHOCK angiographic substudy. *EuroIntervention* **2021**, *16*, e1237–e1244. [CrossRef] [PubMed]
50. Gibson, C.M.; Schomig, A. Coronary and myocardial angiography: Angiographic assessment of both epicardial and myocardial perfusion. *Circulation* **2004**, *109*, 3096–3105. [CrossRef] [PubMed]

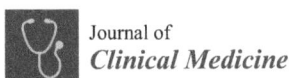

Journal of
Clinical Medicine

Article

Early Detection of Inflammation-Prone STEMI Patients Using the CRP Troponin Test (CTT)

Rafael Y. Brzezinski [1], Ariel Melloul [1], Shlomo Berliner [1], Ilana Goldiner [2], Moshe Stark [2], Ori Rogowski [1], Shmuel Banai [3], Shani Shenhar-Tsarfaty [1] and Yacov Shacham [3,*]

1. Internal Medicine "C", "D", and "E", Tel Aviv Medical Center, Affiliated with the Sackler Faculty of Medicine, Tel Aviv University, Tel Aviv 69978, Israel; brzezinski@mail.tau.ac.il (R.Y.B.); arielme@tlvmc.gov.il (A.M.); berliners@tlvmc.gov.il (S.B.); orir@tlvmc.gov.il (O.R.); shanis@tlvmc.gov.il (S.S.-T.)
2. Department of Clinical Laboratories, Tel Aviv Medical Center, Affiliated with the Sackler Faculty of Medicine, Tel Aviv University, Tel Aviv 69978, Israel; ilanag@tlvmc.gov.il (I.G.); moshes@tlvmc.gov.il (M.S.)
3. Department of Cardiology, Tel Aviv Medical Center, Affiliated with the Sackler Faculty of Medicine, Tel Aviv University, Tel Aviv 69978, Israel; shmuelb@tlvmc.gov.il
* Correspondence: kobys@tlvmc.gov.il

Abstract: Elevated concentrations of C-reactive protein (CRP) early during an acute coronary syndrome (ACS) may reflect the magnitude of the inflammatory response to myocardial damage and are associated with worse outcome. However, the routine measurement of both CRP and cardiac troponin simultaneously in the setting of ST-segment myocardial infarction (STEMI) is not used broadly. Here, we sought to identify and characterize individuals who are prone to an elevated inflammatory response following STEMI by using a combined CRP and troponin test (CTT) and determine their short- and long-term outcome. We retrospectively examined 1186 patients with the diagnosis of acute STEMI, who had at least two successive measurements of combined CRP and cardiac troponin (up to 6 h apart), all within the first 48 h of admission. We used Chi-Square Automatic Interaction Detector (CHΛID) tree analysis to determine which parameters, timing (baseline vs. serial measurements), and cut-offs should be used to predict mortality. Patients with high CRP concentrations (above 90th percentile, >33 mg/L) had higher 30 day and all-cause mortality rates compared to the rest of the cohort, regardless of their troponin test status (above or below 118,000 ng/L); 14.4% vs. 2.7%, $p < 0.01$. Furthermore, patients with both high CRP and high troponin levels on their second measurement had the highest 30-day mortality rates compared to the rest of the cohort; 21.4% vs. 3.7%, $p < 0.01$. These patients also had the highest all-cause mortality rates after a median follow-up of 4.5 years compared to the rest of the cohort; 42.9% vs. 12.7%, $p < 0.01$. In conclusion, serial measurements of both CRP and cardiac troponin might detect patients at increased risk for short-and long-term mortality following STEMI. We suggest the future use of the combined CTT as a potential early marker for inflammatory-prone patients with worse outcomes following ACS. This sub-type of patients might benefit from early anti-inflammatory therapy such as colchicine and anti-interleukin-1ß agents.

Keywords: CRP; troponin; STEMI; acute coronary syndrome; inflammation

Citation: Brzezinski, R.Y.; Melloul, A.; Berliner, S.; Goldiner, I.; Stark, M.; Rogowski, O.; Banai, S.; Shenhar-Tsarfaty, S.; Shacham, Y. Early Detection of Inflammation-Prone STEMI Patients Using the CRP Troponin Test (CTT). J. Clin. Med. 2022, 11, 2453. https://doi.org/10.3390/jcm11092453

Academic Editor: Ahmed Sheriff

Received: 17 March 2022
Accepted: 25 April 2022
Published: 27 April 2022

Publisher's Note: MDPI stays neutral with regard to jurisdictional claims in published maps and institutional affiliations.

Copyright: © 2022 by the authors. Licensee MDPI, Basel, Switzerland. This article is an open access article distributed under the terms and conditions of the Creative Commons Attribution (CC BY) license (https://creativecommons.org/licenses/by/4.0/).

1. Introduction

Cardiac troponin is a sensitive and specific marker for myocardial injury, and its prognostic value in acute coronary syndrome (ACS) is well established [1]. Elevated concentrations of C-reactive protein (CRP) in patients with coronary artery disease (CAD) are associated with atherosclerotic disease activity and worse clinical outcomes [2–5]. Moreover, the rate of increase in CRP levels early after ACS onset is correlated with increased mortality rates and myocardial damage [6–8]. Finally, multivariable risk models have identified cardiac troponin and CRP as significant and independent predictors of risk in patients with ACS, with additive predictive value [5]. Yet, the routine measurement of both CRP and cardiac troponin simultaneously in the setting of ST-segment myocardial infarction (STEMI) is not used broadly and is still not recommended by recent clinical guidelines [9].

Systemic vascular inflammation plays a pivotal role in the progression of CAD, and several anti-inflammatory therapies have been examined in recent trials, including methotrexate [10], anti-interleukin (IL)-1ß [11], and colchicine [12], for the secondary prevention of atherosclerotic cardiovascular disease. However, it seems increased patient variability exists in the extent of the inflammatory response to cardiomyocyte necrosis and the progression of ACS [5]. Thus, more individualized approaches based on circulating inflammatory biomarkers are needed to identify patients who will benefit from these therapies.

Here, we sought to identify individuals who are prone to an elevated inflammatory response following STEMI using serial simultaneous measurements of both CRP and cardiac troponin-I during the first 48 h of admission. We characterized patients based on their CRP-Troponin-Test (CTT) results and determined their short- and long-term outcome.

2. Materials and Methods

2.1. Study Design and Clinical Data

We performed a retrospective, single-center observational study at the Tel-Aviv Sourasky Medical Center. We included consecutive patients admitted between January 2008 and January 2020 to the Cardiac Intensive Care Unit (CICU) with the diagnosis of acute STEMI, who had at least two successive measurements of both CRP and cardiac troponin levels within the first 48 h of admission [6,8]. The CTT result was derived from test findings of a CRP and a troponin measurement carried out up to 6 h apart.

The diagnosis of STEMI was based on a typical history of chest pain, diagnostic electrocardiographic changes, and serial elevation of serum cardiac biomarkers [1]. Primary percutaneous coronary intervention (PCI) was performed in patients with symptoms ≤ 12 h in duration as well as in patients with symptoms lasting 12–24 h if the symptoms continued to persist during hospitalization.

CAD was defined if a $\geq 50\%$ narrowing in an epicardial coronary artery was present, or a history of coronary intervention (stent or angioplasty) to an epicardial coronary artery, or bypass surgery. CAD severity was divided into 4 categories according to the number of diseased vessels (i.e., 0, 1, 2, or 3) as previously described [13,14]. Following primary PCI left ventricular (LV) ejection fraction was measured in all patients by bedside echocardiography, within the first 48 h of admission.

The MDClone platform was used to automatically extract multiple demographic and clinical variables from Electronic Health Records as well as determine 30-day and all-cause mortality rates [15]. Missing data on cardiovascular history, clinical risk factors, treatment characteristics, and laboratory results were manually retrieved from the patients' medical files. The median follow-up time for all-cause mortality was 4.5 years (interquartile range [IQR] 3.1–6.3).

2.2. Laboratory Tests

Complete blood count parameters were measured with a Coulter STKS electronic counter. Blood samples for CRP and cardiac troponin assessments were drawn in all patients upon admission to the emergency department or at the catheterization laboratory prior to primary PCI. A second sample was drawn following primary PCI, and within 48 h from CICU admission.

The white blood count (WBC) was determined by the Coulter STKS (Beckman Coulter, Nyon, Switzerland) electronic cell analyzer. Wide range C-reactive protein (CRP) levels were determined by the Bayer wr-CRP assay (Bayer, Leverkusen, Germany) [16]. High-sensitivity cardiac troponin I was measured by an ADVIA Centaur® TnI-Ultra® assay (Siemens, Munich, Germany).

2.3. Statistical Analysis

All continuous variables are displayed as means (±standard deviation (SD)) for normally distributed variables or median (interquartile range (IQR)) for variables with abnormal distribution. Categorical variables are displayed as numbers (%) of subjects within each group. Continuous variables were compared by a student's *t*-test for normally distributed variables and by the Mann–Whitney U test for non-normally distributed ones. To assess associations among categorical variables, we used a Chi-square test. We assessed normal distributions using Kolmogorov–Smirnov's test and Q-Q plots. The correlations between continuous variables were assessed by Pearson's r for normally distributed variables and Spearmen's r for variables with abnormal distribution.

To determine which CRP and troponin measurements (baseline vs. serial measurements), and corresponding cut-offs should be used to predict 30-day mortality, we used Chi-square automatic interaction detection (CHAID) [17]. CHAID analysis builds a predictive model to determine the best cutoffs for the input variables to predict an outcome. In CHAID, continuous predictors are split into categories with an approximately equal number of observations. CHAID creates all possible cross-tabulations for each categorical predictor until the best outcome is achieved and no further splitting can be performed. Patients were divided into groups according to the output cutoffs.

To adjust for possible confounding variables, we used a binary logistic regression to predict 30-day mortality status. We adjusted our model for the combined second CTT test status, age, sex, and conventional risk factors including history of heart failure, prior myocardial infarction (MI), diabetes, hypertension, and hyperlipidemia. Adjusted odds ratios (OR) with 95% confidence intervals (CI) were reported.

A two-tailed $p < 0.05$ was considered statistically significant. All analyses were performed with the SPSS (IBM SPSS Statistics, version 28, IBM Corp., Armonk, NY, USA, 2016) and GraphPad Prism version 9.00 (GraphPad Software, La Jolla, CA, USA).

3. Results

3.1. Patient Characteristics

Patient characteristics are displayed in Table 1. The final study cohort included 1186 STEMI patients. The mean age was 63.2 ± 13 years, and 207 patients (17.5%) were women. The distribution of the second CTT test results is presented in Figure 1.

The median first and second CRP levels were 4.3 [IQR 1.5–11.1] and 5 [IQR 1.6–11.8] mg/L, respectively. The corresponding median first and second troponin levels were 430.5 [64.7–4967.5] and 9995.5 [1778.7–43,631.7] ng/L. The correlation between CRP and cardiac troponin was $r = 0.28$ for the first measurement, and $r = 0.22$ for the second measurement, $p < 0.01$ for both. Notably, the correlation between the first troponin and the second CRP was stronger ($r = 0.37$, $p < 0.01$) and might reflect the slower rate of CRP increase compared to cardiac troponin following myocardial infarction [18].

A total of 46 patients (3.9%) died within 30 days of admission (mean age = 80.3 ± 10 years). We used CHAID tree analysis to determine which CTT measurement and cutoffs should be used to predict 30-day mortality. A second CRP level > 33 mg/L (90th percentile of the cohort) was associated with the highest 30-day mortality rate. Accordingly, patients were divided into four groups based on their combined CTT results, i.e., CRP/troponin levels above or below the 90th percentile (Figure 1 and Table 1).

Patients with both high CRP (>33 mg/L) and high troponin (>118,000 ng/L) levels were older and had a higher prevalence of diabetes mellitus and prior heart failure compared to the rest of the cohort (Table 1). Individuals with high CRP levels had a higher prevalence of hypertension, regardless of their troponin test result (Table 1). Of note, the severity of CAD was similar across all groups.

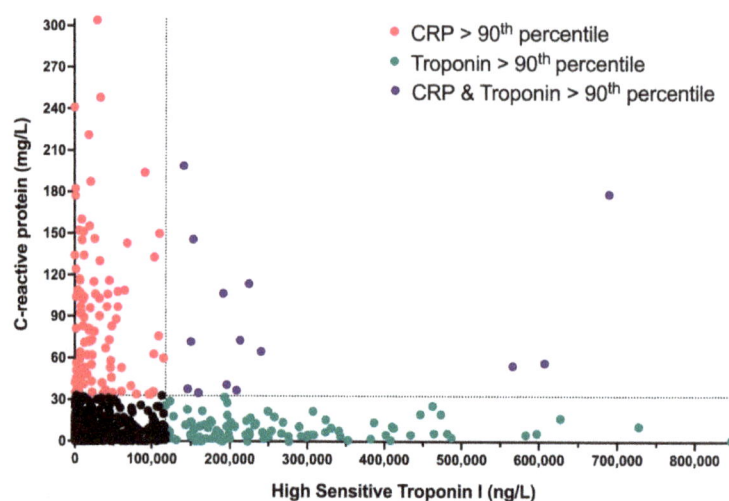

Figure 1. Combined CRP and Troponin Test (CTT) results. A scatterplot of the study population according to their second CRP and cardiac troponin test results. The dotted lines represent the 90th percentile thresholds (CRP > 33 mg/L and cardiac troponin > 118,000 ng/L) according to our CHIAD analysis as described in the Methods section.

Table 1. Baseline clinical characteristics by CTT * results (total n = 1186).

	CRP < 90th Percentile (<33 mg/L)		CRP > 90th Percentile (>33 mg/L)		p-Value
	Trop < 90th %ile (<118,000 ng/L)	Trop > 90th %ile (>118,000 ng/L)	Trop < 90th %ile (<118,000 ng/L)	Trop > 90th %ile (>118,000 ng/L)	
n	964	104	104	14	
Age, years (±SD)	62.6 (12.9)	62.9 (13.9)	67.9 (14.5)	68.0 (15.4)	<0.01
Women, n (%)	176 (18)	8 (8)	22 (21)	1 (7)	0.03
Ejection fraction, % (±SD)	38.3 (19.6)	32.9 (16.6)	33.8 (19.6)	27.9 (16.5)	<0.01
Diabetes, n (%)	243 (25)	18 (17)	43 (41)	7 (50)	<0.01
History of HF, n (%)	95 (10)	22 (21)	25 (24)	8 (57)	<0.01
Past MI, n (%)	174 18.1	19 (18.3)	28 (27)	1 (7.1)	0.11
Hyperlipidemia, n (%)	499 (52)	46 (44)	59 (57)	10 (71)	0.13
Current smoker, n (%)	466 (49)	55 (54)	44 (44)	3 (23)	0.13
Hypertension, n (%)	449 (47)	39 (38)	61 (59)	7 (50)	0.02
CAD severity					0.11
0 diseased vessels, n (%)	6 (1)	0 (0)	1 (1)	0 (0)	
1 diseased vessel, n (%)	378 (40)	46 (44)	32 (33)	2 (15)	
2 diseased vessels, n (%)	313 (33)	31 (30)	24 (25)	7 (54)	
3 diseased vessels, n (%)	255 (27)	27 (26)	39 (41)	4 (31)	
Glucose, mg/dL (±SD)	150.3 (60.8)	154.5 (67.0)	170.7 (89.5)	220.7 (109.3)	<0.01
HbA1C, % (±SD)	5.9 [5.6, 6.5]	5.8 [5.5, 6.3]	6.0 [5.7, 7.1]	5.8 [5.7, 6.5]	0.15
WBC, 10^9/L (±SD)	11.8 (4.2)	13.4 (3.8)	12.6 (4.3)	14.9 (5.2)	<0.01
1st CRP, mg/L [IQR]	3.5 [1.3, 8.2]	4.2 [1.4, 7.8]	58.0 [43.1, 109.8]	66.6 [25.5, 119.9]	<0.01
2nd CRP, mg/L [IQR]	3.9 [1.4, 8.8]	5.8 [2.9, 12.6]	72.7 [45.3, 108.7]	68.8 [44.3, 112.3]	<0.01
1st Troponin, ng/L [IQR]	299.5 [48.0, 2618.8]	6021.5 [137.0, 54,233.2]	8127.5 [1770.0, 23,908.5]	33,484.0 [7278.2, 125,331.0]	<0.01
2nd Troponin, ng/L [IQR])	6689.0 [1192.0, 23,949.8]	222,112.0 [174,063.8, 307,510.2]	18,453.5 [6795.0, 42,399.5]	202,177.0 [154,482.0, 236,586.5]	<0.01

* CTT—CRP Troponin Test (second measurement); CRP—C-Reactive Protein; HbA1c—Hemoglobin A1c; HF—Heart Failure; MI—Myocardial Infarction; PLT—Platelets; Trop—Cardiac Troponin I; WBC—White Blood Count.

3.2. CTT Results and 30-Day/All-Cause Mortality

Patients with high CRP concentrations (above the 90th percentile, >33mg/L) had higher 30-day and all-cause mortality rates regardless of their troponin test status (above or below 118,000 ng/L); 14.4% vs. 2.7%, $p < 0.01$ (Figure 2). However, patients with both high CRP and high troponin levels had the highest mortality rates compared to the rest of the cohort; 21.4% vs. 3.7%, $p < 0.01$ (Figure 2). We also assessed all-cause mortality after a median follow-up of 4.5 years [IQR 3.1–6.3] and observed a similar trend across all CTT test result categories (Figure 2). Patients with both high CRP and high troponin levels on their second measurement had the highest mortality rates compared to the rest of the cohort; 42.9% vs. 12.7%, $p < 0.01$ (Figure 2).

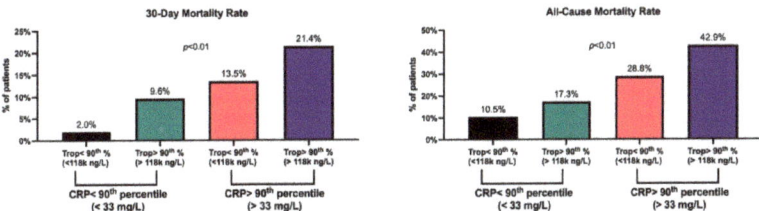

Figure 2. Combined CRP and Troponin Test (CTT) results and mortality rates. Bar graphs representing the proportion of patients who died during follow-up according to their CRP Troponin Test (CTT) results. The median follow-up time for all-cause mortality was 4.5 years [IQR 3.1–6.3]. The bar colors correspond to the 4 groups presented in Figure 1. *p*-values were calculated by the Chi-Square test.

Finally, a binary logistic regression analysis showed that the combined result of the second CTT significantly predicted 30-day mortality after adjusting for age, sex, and conventional risk factors; OR = 6.98 95% CI 1.4, 35.5, $p = 0.02$ for patients with both high CRP and high troponin on their second measurement (above 90th percentile). Age and a history of heart failure were also significant predictors in the model (Table 2).

Table 2. Binary logistic regression to predict 30-day mortality.

	Odds Ratio	95.0% CI		*p* Value
		Lower	Upper	
Age (years)	1.092	1.053	1.132	<0.01
Sex (women)	1.825	0.787	4.233	0.16
Diabetes mellitus	1.993	0.935	4.246	0.07
History of HF	10.914	5.201	22.903	<0.01
Past MI	0.896	0.387	2.078	0.79
Hyperlipidemia	1.320	0.584	2.984	0.5
Hypertension	1.451	0.578	3.642	0.43
2nd CTT result (normal CRP and troponin as indicator)				
High troponin-normal CRP	6.896	2.531	18.788	<0.01
Normal troponin-high CRP	4.756	1.960	11.543	<0.01
High troponin-high CRP	6.974	1.372	35.457	0.02

Method = Enter. CTT—CRP Troponin Test (second measurement); CRP—C-Reactive Protein; HF—Heart Failure.

4. Discussion

The main findings of our study are that serial simultaneous measurements of cardiac troponin and CRP within the first 48 h of admission might identify patients at increased risk for short- and long-term mortality following STEMI. Patients with both high CRP and high troponin levels (above 90th percentile) were at increased risk for 30-day and all-cause mortality during a median follow-up of 4.5 years. We propose here the use of the combined CTT as an early and simple marker for inflammatory-prone patients with worse outcomes following ACS.

Our results portray the wide spectrum of the human inflammatory response to MI by considering cardiac troponin as the "antigen" in this relatively sterile inflammatory process. We show that some individuals demonstrate low systemic inflammation (evidenced by low CRP levels) even in the presence of extremely high myocardial necrosis (cardiac troponin > 118,000 ng/L) (Figure 1). On the other hand, some individuals with very low levels of troponin had extremely high CRP levels (>33 mg/L) and appear to be more "inflammatory prone" to myocardial necrosis. These inflammatory-prone patients had increased 30-day and long-term mortality rates. Moreover, our findings show that patients with elevated levels of CRP during STEMI have higher mortality rates regardless of their troponin levels on presentation (Figure 2). These results are in line with several past reports on the prognostic value of CRP in ACS [2,19–24]. Our findings are also in line with existing reports on the association between CRP levels and infarct size in STEMI patients, as well as the development of cardiac remodeling and microvascular disease during follow-up [25–29]. The cutoffs for "high" CRP in these reports ranged from 20–40 mg/L and are relatively similar to the ones used in our analysis. The higher mortality rates of patients with both high CRP and high troponin could be explained by the higher prevalence of heart failure and diabetes among these individuals. Nonetheless, it is reasonable to speculate that their inflammatory-prone nature played a major part in the development of these existing comorbidities in the first place, and thereby underline the importance of our findings.

Recent studies have suggested that serial CRP measurements can help reclassify stable and unstable CAD patients undergoing coronary interventions by assessing their "residual inflammatory risk" in terms of long-term outcomes [5,21,30,31]. The time interval between CRP measurements in these reports was around 4 weeks. Others have suggested a combined approach of multiple inflammatory biomarkers for improved risk stratification during STEMI [23,24,27,32]. Moreover, we and others have demonstrated that CRP velocity between two serial measurements within the first days of hospitalization is associated with increased mortality, left ventricular dysfunction, microvascular damage, and acute kidney injury [6,7,33,34]. We suggest here the addition of high sensitivity cardiac troponin to CRP across all time points to further improve risk stratification of CAD patients that underwent a coronary intervention. Most importantly, the CTT could be used to identify the precise subtype of patients that might benefit from early anti-inflammatory therapy, such as colchicine [12] and anti-IL-1ß agents [30]. We hypothesize that our "inflammatory-prone" patients who had high CRP levels—even in the presence of relatively low or normal troponin levels—are the ones who are most likely to benefit from these treatments.

Our study has several limitations. First, the retrospective nature of this study and the non-standardized timing of both CRP and troponin measurements poses a risk of residual confounding. Furthermore, the maximum time interval between the first and second CTTs was arbitrarily set at 48 h from admission. Future standardized, large-scale efforts are needed to determine the optimal time intervals between serial measurements. Finally, the cutoffs for both CRP and troponin levels used here were optimized for this specific study sample and may not present the same diagnostic yield in other populations. Moreover, the relatively small group of patients with both high CRP and troponin ($n = 14$) limits the statistical power of additional analyses aimed to detect residual confounding. Future studies should evaluate these cutoffs in other non-Caucasian populations and also explore the possibility of sex-specific thresholds [35]. Furthermore, large-scale studies should stratify patients according to pre-existing comorbidities, especially heart failure, in their analysis to possibly define specific thresholds for these patients.

In summary, we suggest further investigation of the novel CTT as an early clinical assessment tool for identifying patients at increased risk for worse outcome following STEMI. Future clinical trials should investigate the usefulness of the CTT in improving optimal patient selection to receive novel anti-inflammatory agents in the setting of ACS.

Author Contributions: Conceptualization, S.B. (Shlomo Berliner), S.S.-T. and Y.S.; data curation, R.Y.B., S.S.-T. and Y.S.; formal analysis, R.Y.B., A.M. and S.S.-T.; funding acquisition, S.B. (Shlomo Berliner), S.S.-T. and Y.S.; investigation, R.Y.B., A.M., S.S.-T. and Y.S.; methodology, R.Y.B., A.M., I.G., M.S. and S.S.-T.; project administration, O.R. and S.S.-T.; resources, S.B. (Shlomo Berliner), I.G., M.S., O.R., S.B. (Shmuel Banai) and Y.S.; software, R.Y.B. and A.M.; supervision, S.B. (Shlomo Berliner), O.R., S.B. (Shmuel Banai), S.S.-T. and Y.S.; validation, O.R.; writing—original draft, R.Y.B. and S.S.-T.; writing—review and editing, R.Y.B., S.B. (Shlomo Berliner), S.B. (Shmuel Banai), S.S.-T. and Y.S. All authors have read and agreed to the published version of the manuscript.

Funding: This research received no external funding.

Institutional Review Board Statement: The study was conducted in accordance with the Declaration of Helsinki and was approved by the Tel-Aviv Sourasky Medical Center Institutional Review Board (Study number: TLV-16-0224).

Informed Consent Statement: Informed consent was obtained from all subjects involved in this study.

Data Availability Statement: Data will be made available upon reasonable request.

Acknowledgments: We thank Eyal Egoz and Liran Harel for their help with the MDClone big data platform.

Conflicts of Interest: The authors declare no conflict of interest.

References

1. Thygesen, K.; Alpert, J.S.; Jaffe, A.S.; Chaitman, B.R.; Bax, J.J.; Morrow, D.A.; White, H.D.; Mickley, H.; Crea, F.; Van De Werf, F.; et al. Fourth universal definition of myocardial infarction (2018). *Eur. Heart J.* **2019**, *40*, 237–269. [CrossRef] [PubMed]
2. Yip, H.K.; Hang, C.L.; Fang, C.Y.; Hsieh, Y.K.; Yang, C.H.; Hung, W.C.; Wu, C.J. Level of high-sensitivity C-reactive protein is predictive of 30-day outcomes in patients with acute myocardial infarction undergoing primary coronary intervention. *Chest* **2005**, *127*, 803–808. [CrossRef] [PubMed]
3. De Winter, R.J.; Heyde, G.S.; Koch, K.T.; Fischer, J.; Van Straalen, J.P.; Bax, M.; Schotborgh, C.E.; Mulder, K.J.; Sanders, G.T.; Piek, J.J.; et al. The prognostic value of pre-procedural plasma C-reactive protein in patients undergoing elective coronary angioplasty. *Eur. Heart J.* **2002**, *23*, 960–966. [CrossRef] [PubMed]
4. Arroyo-Espliguero, R.; Avanzas, P.; Cosín-Sales, J.; Aldama, G.; Pizzi, C.; Kaski, J.C. C-reactive protein elevation and disease activity in patients with coronary artery disease. *Eur. Heart J.* **2004**, *25*, 401–408. [CrossRef]
5. Lawler, P.R.; Bhatt, D.L.; Godoy, L.C.; Lüscher, T.F.; Bonow, R.O.; Verma, S.; Ridker, P.M. Targeting cardiovascular inflammation: Next steps in clinical translation. *Eur. Heart J.* **2021**, *42*, 113–131. [CrossRef]
6. Milwidsky, A.; Ziv-Baran, T.; Letourneau-Shesaf, S.; Keren, G.; Taieb, P.; Berliner, S.; Shacham, Y. CRP velocity and short-term mortality in ST segment elevation myocardial infarction. *Biomarkers* **2017**, *22*, 383–386. [CrossRef]
7. Holzknecht, M.; Tiller, C.; Reindl, M.; Lechner, I.; Fink, P.; Lunger, P.; Mayr, A.; Henninger, B.; Brenner, C.; Klug, G.; et al. Association of C-Reactive Protein Velocity with Early Left Ventricular Dysfunction in Patients with First ST-Elevation Myocardial Infarction. *J. Clin. Med.* **2021**, *10*, 5494. [CrossRef]
8. Banai, A.; Levit, D.; Morgan, S.; Loewenstein, I.; Merdler, I.; Hochstadt, A.; Szekely, Y.; Topilsky, Y.; Banai, S.; Shacham, Y. Association between C-Reactive Protein Velocity and Left Ventricular Function in Patients with ST-Elevated Myocardial Infarction. *J. Clin. Med.* **2022**, *11*, 401. [CrossRef]
9. Ibanez, B.; James, S.; Agewall, S.; Antunes, M.J.; Bucciarelli-Ducci, C.; Bueno, H.; Caforio, A.L.P.; Crea, F.; Goudevenos, J.A.; Halvorsen, S.; et al. 2017 ESC Guidelines for the management of acute myocardial infarction in patients presenting with ST-segment elevationThe Task Force for the management of acute myocardial infarction in patients presenting with ST-segment elevation of the European Society of Cardiology (ESC). *Eur. Heart J.* **2018**, *39*, 119–177. [CrossRef]
10. Ridker, P.M.; Everett, B.M.; Pradhan, A.; MacFadyen, J.G.; Solomon, D.H.; Zaharris, E.; Mam, V.; Hasan, A.; Rosenberg, Y.; Iturriaga, E.; et al. Low-Dose Methotrexate for the Prevention of Atherosclerotic Events. *N. Engl. J. Med.* **2019**, *380*, 752–762. [CrossRef]
11. Ridker, P.M.; Everett, B.M.; Thuren, T.; MacFadyen, J.G.; Chang, W.H.; Ballantyne, C.; Fonseca, F.; Nicolau, J.; Koenig, W.; Anker, S.D.; et al. Antiinflammatory Therapy with Canakinumab for Atherosclerotic Disease. *N. Engl. J. Med.* **2017**, *377*, 1119–1131. [CrossRef]
12. Tardif, J.-C.; Kouz, S.; Waters, D.D.; Bertrand, O.F.; Diaz, R.; Maggioni, A.P.; Pinto, F.J.; Ibrahim, R.; Gamra, H.; Kiwan, G.S.; et al. Efficacy and Safety of Low-Dose Colchicine after Myocardial Infarction. *N. Engl. J. Med.* **2019**, *381*, 2497–2505. [CrossRef]
13. Arbel, Y.; Finkelstein, A.; Halkin, A.; Birati, E.Y.; Revivo, M.; Zuzut, M.; Shevach, A.; Berliner, S.; Herz, I.; Keren, G.; et al. Neutrophil/lymphocyte ratio is related to the severity of coronary artery disease and clinical outcome in patients undergoing angiography. *Atherosclerosis* **2012**, *225*, 456–460. [CrossRef]

14. Mohr, F.W.; Morice, M.C.; Kappetein, A.P.; Feldman, T.E.; Ståhle, E.; Colombo, A.; MacK, M.J.; Holmes, D.R.; Morel, M.A.; Van Dyck, N.; et al. Coronary artery bypass graft surgery versus percutaneous coronary intervention in patients with three-vessel disease and left main coronary disease: 5-year follow-up of the randomised, clinical SYNTAX trial. *Lancet* **2013**, *381*, 629–638. [CrossRef]
15. Reiner Benaim, A.; Almog, R.; Gorelik, Y.; Hochberg, I.; Nassar, L.; Mashiach, T.; Khamaisi, M.; Lurie, Y.; Azzam, Z.S.; Khoury, J.; et al. Analyzing Medical Research Results Based on Synthetic Data and Their Relation to Real Data Results: Systematic Comparison From Five Observational Studies. *JMIR Med. Inform.* **2020**, *8*, e16492. [CrossRef]
16. Arbel, Y.; Eros, Y.; Rogowski, O.; Berliner, S.; Shapira, I.; Keren, G.; Vered, Y.; Banai, S. Comparison of Values of Wide-Range C-Reactive Protein to High-Sensitivity C-Reactive Protein in Patients Undergoing Coronary Angiography. *Am. J. Cardiol.* **2007**, *99*, 1504–1506. [CrossRef]
17. Magidson, J.; SPPS, Inc. *SPSS for Windows, CHAID, Release 6.0*; SPSS: Chicago, IL, USA, 1993; ISBN 0131788493 9780131788497.
18. Townsend, M.J.; Monroe, J.G.; Chan, A.C. B-cell targeted therapies in human autoimmune diseases: An updated perspective. *Immunol. Rev.* **2010**, *237*, 264–283. [CrossRef]
19. Ortolani, P.; Marzocchi, A.; Marrozzini, C.; Palmerini, T.; Saia, F.; Taglieri, N.; Baldazzi, F.; Silenzi, S.; Bacchi-Reggiani, M.L.; Guastaroba, P.; et al. Predictive value of high sensitivity C-reactive protein in patients with ST-elevation myocardial infarction treated with percutaneous coronary intervention. *Eur. Heart J.* **2008**, *29*, 1241–1249. [CrossRef]
20. Théroux, P.; Armstrong, P.W.; Mahaffey, K.W.; Hochman, J.S.; Malloy, K.J.; Rollins, S.; Nicolau, J.C.; Lavoie, J.; The, M.L.; Burchenal, J.; et al. Prognostic significance of blood markers of inflammation in patients with ST-segment elevation myocardial infarction undergoing primary angioplasty and effects of pexelizumab, a C5 inhibitor: A substudy of the COMMA trial. *Eur. Heart J.* **2005**, *26*, 1964–1970. [CrossRef]
21. Kalkman, D.N.; Aquino, M.; Claessen, B.E.; Baber, U.; Guedeney, P.; Sorrentino, S.; Vogel, B.; De Winter, R.J.; Sweeny, J.; Kovacic, J.C.; et al. Residual inflammatory risk and the impact on clinical outcomes in patients after percutaneous coronary interventions. *Eur. Heart J.* **2018**, *39*, 4101–4108. [CrossRef]
22. Tiller, C.; Reindl, M.; Holzknecht, M.; Lechner, I.; Simma, F.; Schwaiger, J.; Mayr, A.; Klug, G.; Bauer, A.; Reinstadler, S.J.; et al. High sensitivity C-reactive protein is associated with worse infarct healing after revascularized ST-elevation myocardial infarction. *Int. J. Cardiol.* **2021**, *328*, 191–196. [CrossRef]
23. Feistritzer, H.-J.; Reinstadler, S.J.; Klug, G.; Reindl, M.; Wöhrer, S.; Brenner, C.; Mayr, A.; Mair, J.; Metzler, B. Multimarker approach for the prediction of microvascular obstruction after acute ST-segment elevation myocardial infarction: A prospective, observational study. *BMC Cardiovasc. Disord.* **2016**, *16*, 239. [CrossRef]
24. Reinstadler, S.J.; Feistritzer, H.J.; Reindl, M.; Klug, G.; Mayr, A.; Mair, J.; Jaschke, W.; Metzler, B. Combined biomarker testing for the prediction of left ventricular remodelling in ST-elevation myocardial infarction. *Open Hear.* **2016**, *3*, e000485. [CrossRef]
25. Ries, W.; Torzewski, J.; Heigl, F.; Pfluecke, C.; Kelle, S.; Darius, H.; Ince, H.; Mitzner, S.; Nordbeck, P.; Butter, C.; et al. C-Reactive Protein Apheresis as Anti-inflammatory Therapy in Acute Myocardial Infarction: Results of the CAMI-1 Study. *Front. Cardiovasc. Med.* **2021**, *8*, 591714. [CrossRef]
26. Reinstadler, S.J.; Kronbichler, A.; Reindl, M.; Feistritzer, H.J.; Innerhofer, V.; Mayr, A.; Klug, G.; Tiefenthaler, M.; Mayer, G.; Metzler, B. Acute kidney injury is associated with microvascular myocardial damage following myocardial infarction. *Kidney Int.* **2017**, *92*, 743–750. [CrossRef]
27. Reindl, M.; Reinstadler, S.J.; Feistritzer, H.J.; Klug, G.; Tiller, C.; Mair, J.; Mayr, A.; Jaschke, W.; Metzler, B. Relation of inflammatory markers with myocardial and microvascular injury in patients with reperfused ST-elevation myocardial infarction. *Eur. Hear. J. Acute Cardiovasc. Care* **2017**, *6*, 640–649. [CrossRef]
28. Reindl, M.; Tiller, C.; Holzknecht, M.; Lechner, I.; Henninger, B.; Mayr, A.; Brenner, C.; Klug, G.; Bauer, A.; Metzler, B.; et al. Association of Myocardial Injury With Serum Procalcitonin Levels in Patients With ST-Elevation Myocardial Infarction. *JAMA Netw. Open* **2020**, *3*, e207030. [CrossRef] [PubMed]
29. Vanhaverbeke, M.; Veltman, D.; Pattyn, N.; De Crem, N.; Gilijns, H.; Cornelissen, V.; Janssens, S.; Sinnaeve, P.R. C-reactive protein during and after myocardial infarction in relation to cardiac injury and left ventricular function at follow-up. *Clin. Cardiol.* **2018**, *41*, 1201–1206. [CrossRef] [PubMed]
30. Ridker, P.M.; MacFadyen, J.G.; Everett, B.M.; Libby, P.; Thuren, T.; Glynn, R.J.; Kastelein, J.; Koenig, W.; Genest, J.; Lorenzatti, A.; et al. Relationship of C-reactive protein reduction to cardiovascular event reduction following treatment with canakinumab: A secondary analysis from the CANTOS randomised controlled trial. *Lancet* **2018**, *391*, 319–328. [CrossRef]
31. Candreva, A.; Matter, C.M. Is the amount of glow predicting the fire? Residual inflammatory risk after percutaneous coronary intervention. *Eur. Heart J.* **2022**, *43*, e10–e13. [CrossRef] [PubMed]
32. Reindl, M.; Reinstadler, S.J.; Feistritzer, H.J.; Mueller, L.; Koch, C.; Mayr, A.; Theurl, M.; Kirchmair, R.; Klug, G.; Metzler, B. Fibroblast growth factor 23 as novel biomarker for early risk stratification after ST-elevation myocardial infarction. *Heart* **2017**, *103*, 856–862. [CrossRef]
33. Holzknecht, M.; Tiller, C.; Reindl, M.; Lechner, I.; Troger, F.; Hosp, M.; Mayr, A.; Brenner, C.; Klug, G.; Bauer, A.; et al. C-reactive protein velocity predicts microvascular pathology after acute ST-elevation myocardial infarction. *Int. J. Cardiol.* **2021**, *338*, 30–36. [CrossRef]

34. Zahler, D.; Rozenfeld, K.L.; Stein, M.; Milwidsky, A.; Berliner, S.; Banai, S.; Arbel, Y.; Shacham, Y. C-reactive protein velocity and the risk of acute kidney injury among ST elevation myocardial infarction patients undergoing primary percutaneous intervention. *J. Nephrol.* **2019**, *32*, 437–443. [CrossRef]
35. Lee, K.K.; Ferry, A.V.; Lee, K.K.; Chapman, A.R.; Sandeman, D.; Adamson, P.D.; Stables, C.L.; Berry, C.; Tsanasis, A.; Marshall, L.; et al. Sex-Specific Thresholds of High-Sensitivity Troponin in Patients With Suspected Acute Coronary Syndrome. *J. Am. Coll. Cardiol.* **2019**, *74*, 2032–2043. [CrossRef]

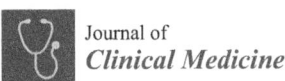

Article

Sepsis Related Mortality Associated with an Inflammatory Burst in Patients Admitting to the Department of Internal Medicine with Apparently Normal C-Reactive Protein Concentration

Ronnie Meilik [1], Hadas Ben-Assayag [1], Ahuva Meilik [2], Shlomo Berliner [1], David Zeltser [1], Itzhak Shapira [1], Ori Rogowski [1], Ilana Goldiner [3], Shani Shenhar-Tsarfaty [1,*] and Asaf Wasserman [1]

[1] Department of Internal Medicine "C", "D", & "E", Tel Aviv Medical Center, Sackler Faculty of Medicine, Tel Aviv University, Tel Aviv 64239, Israel; ronniemeilik@gmail.com (R.M.); hadasba@tlvmc.gov.il (H.B.-A.); berliners@tlvmc.gov.il (S.B.); dzeltser@tlvmc.gov.il (D.Z.); shapira@tlvmc.gov.il (I.S.); orir@tlvmc.gov.il (O.R.); asafw@tlvmc.gov.il (A.W.)
[2] Clinical Performances Research and Operational Unit, Tel Aviv Medical Center, Sackler Faculty of Medicine, Tel Aviv University, Tel Aviv 64239, Israel; ahuvawm@tlvmc.gov.il
[3] Laboratory Medicine, Tel Aviv Medical Center, Sackler Faculty of Medicine, Tel Aviv University, Tel Aviv 64239, Israel; ilanag@tlvmc.gov.il
* Correspondence: shanis@tlvmc.gov.il

Abstract: Background: Patients who are admitted to the Department of Internal Medicine with apparently normal C-reactive protein (CRP) concentration impose a special challenge due to the assumption that they might not harbor a severe and potentially lethal medical condition. Methods: A retrospective cohort of all patients who were admitted to the Department of Internal Medicine with a CRP concentration of ≤ 31.9 mg/L and had a second CRP test obtained within the next 24 h. Seven day mortality data were analyzed. Results: Overall, 3504 patients were analyzed with a mean first and second CRP of 8.8 (8.5) and 14.6 (21.6) mg/L, respectively. The seven day mortality increased from 1.8% in the first quartile of the first CRP to 7.5% in the fourth quartile of the first CRP ($p < 0.0001$) and from 0.6% in the first quartile of the second CRP to 9.5% in the fourth quartile of the second CRP test ($p < 0.0001$), suggesting a clear relation between the admission CRP and in hospital seven day mortality. Conclusions: An association exists between the quartiles of CRP and 7-day mortality as well as sepsis related cause of death. Furthermore, the CRP values 24 h after hospital admission improved the discrimination.

Keywords: C-reactive protein; inflammation; mortality causes

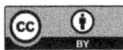

1. Introduction

The admission of patients to the Department of Internal Medicine with apparently normal C-reactive protein (CRP) concentration is a clinical challenge due to the possibility that clinicians might assume that these patients do not harbor a significant inflammatory response. However, the inflammatory response could burst-in later. "Inflammatory burst" is the rapid release of pro-inflammatory cytokines/mediators. Previous studies have shown that any inflammatory process could put the patient at great risk due to tissue damage or necrosis mechanisms [1,2]. Therefore, repeated measures of inflammatory biomarkers are more informative than looking at a single snapshot. We have recently shown that patients who are admitted with very low CRP concentrations do not necessarily present a benign course of their disease [3]. In addition, we could show that a follow-up CRP test could add significant prognostic information to the medical team [4–8]. In fact, a second CRP test could single out those individuals who are at an increased risk of death during hospitalization [9].

We conducted a retrospective study in a cohort of patients who were admitted to the Departments of Internal Medicine with apparently normal C-reactive protein concentration, in whom, a short-term follow-up CRP test was performed. The specific aim of this study was to determine the relation of 7-day mortality to the CRP values in the first 24 h after admission. This information is relevant for the usefulness of doing a follow-up CRP in individuals in whom the treating physician might have an impression of a non-alarming medical condition.

2. Patients, Controls and Methods

2.1. The Patients

We used the MDClone system to retrieve information regarding the patients who were admitted to one of our nine Departments of Internal Medicine at the Tel-Aviv Sourasky Medical Center, a tertiary 1050-bed university affiliated medical center serving a population of about 500,000 residents of the city of Tel-Aviv, Israel. Included were patients who presented with a CRP concentration of ≤ 31.9 mg/L and had a second CRP test obtained within 24 h thereafter. Since no postmortem sections were performed in those individuals who did not survive the first week of hospitalization, the medical records of those patients were manually reviewed on an individual basis in order to determine the presumed cause of death in an as accurate a way as possible.

2.2. The Method to Determine the CRP Cutoff

The method of determining the cutoff CRP concentration was based on data that were available in the Tel-Aviv Medical Center Inflammation Survey (TAMCIS) as previously described [10]. In brief, a CRP concentration of 31.9 mg/L was actually the upper limit of a mean CRP + three S.D. obtained from 17,214 apparently healthy individuals who participated in our health-screening program [11–14]. Therefore, only hospitalized patients with the first CRP measured to be lower or equal to 31.9 mg/L were presently included.

2.3. The MDClone System

Data were retrieved using MDClone (mdclone.com), a query tool that provides the comprehensive patient-level data of wide-ranging variables in a defined period around an index event. Data were collected for all patients over 18 years old hospitalized between June 2007 and September 2020.

2.4. Laboratory Methods

Wide-range CRP (wrCRP) was measured by ADVIA 2400 Siemens Healthcare Diagnostics Inc., Tarrytown, NY 10591-5097 USA using a Latex enhanced immunoturbidimetric method [15].

2.5. Review of Death Causes

Cause of death was determined by reviewing individual record files. After a patient's death, the treating medical team had thoroughly recorded their diagnosis by relying on different findings and the patient's clinical picture during hospitalization. Sepsis, in particularly, was determined as the cause of death when the patients presented with multiorgan failure including shock and cause of death in a picture implying sepsis.

2.6. Statistical Methods

Categorical variables were reported as numbers and percentages. Continuous variables were evaluated for normal distribution and reported as the mean and standard deviation (SD) or as the median and interquartile range (IQR). Subgroup analysis of the first and second CRP levels was conducted using the Mann–Whitney test. The chi squared test or Fishers' exact test were used to compare the categorical variables among patients who survived the first 7 days of admission and those who did not. The receiver operating characteristic (ROC) curve analysis was used to evaluate the serial CRP measurements as the predictor of 7 day mortality. A time-dependent COX regression was used to evaluate the association between each of the CRP measurements and in-hospital mortality. Age, sex, and either the first or second CRP measurements were included in the analysis. A two-tailed p-value < 0.05 was considered as statistically significant. IBM SPSS (IBM Corp. Released 2013. IBM SPSS Statistics for Windows, Version 25.0. Armonk, NY: IBM Corp.) was used for all statistical analyses.

2.7. Ethics Committee Approval

The Tel-Aviv Sourasky Medical Center Institutional Review Board (0491-17-TLV) approved the study.

3. Results

Overall, 3504 inpatients met the inclusion criteria. The mean age was 64.3 (18.5) years. The mean first and second measurements of CRP were 8.8 (8.5) and 14.6 (21.6) mg/L, respectively. The characteristics of the patients are described in Table 1.

Table 1. The characteristics of the patients.

Total Population	N = 3504
Gender (% of males)	1.7
Age (Years: mean ± SD)	64.3 ± 18.5
Hypertension, %	26.7
Diabetes, %	14.4
Ischemic heart disease, %	13.1
Dyslipidemia, %	11.3
CVA %	2.9

CRP is known to be affected by a various factors, therefore, subgroup analysis of the first and second CRP levels was conducted (Table 2). Female gender, diabetes mellitus, hypertension, and ischemic heart disease were associated with higher levels of both the first and second CRP measurements in our cohort.

Table 2. The subgroup analysis of the first and second CRP measurements.

Factor	First CRP (Median, IQR)			Second CRP (Median, IQR)		
	With	Without	p Value	With	Without	p Value
Gender, (Female)	6.24 (1.6–14.0)	5.37 (1.4–13.8)	<0.001	8.45 (2.3–19.5)	7.74 (2.0–19.3)	<0.001
Diabetes Mellitus	7.54 (2.4–15.7)	5.50 (1.3–13.8)	<0.001	9.48 (3.2–20.2)	7.8 (2.0–19.3)	<0.001
Hypertension	6.91 (2.-15.0)	5.38 (1.3–13.8)	<0.001	9.09 (2.9–19.9)	7.7 (1.9–7.7)	<0.001
Dyslipidemia	5.57 (1.7–13.2)	5.81 (1.4–14.3)	0.684	7.47 (2.3–17.6)	8.15 (2.1–19.7)	<0.001
Ischemic heart disease	6.65 (1.9–14.9)	5.66 (1.4–14.0)	<0.001	8.42 (2.4–19.3)	8.02 (2.1–19.4)	0.008

In Table 3, we present the results of the first CRP divided into quartiles. It can be seen that the seven day mortality rates increased from 1.7% in the first CRP quartile to 7.8% in the fourth one (chi-square statistics was 37.6, $p < 0.0001$).

Table 3. The number of patients who died within 7 days according to the quartiles of the first and second CRP measurements.

	First CRP Measurement					Second CRP Measurement			
Quartile	n	CRP, mg/L	Deaths within 7 Days n, (%)	Sepsis Related Deaths, n, (%)	Quartile	n	CRP, mg/L	Deaths within 7 Days n, (%)	Sepsis Related Deaths, n, (%)
1	878	0.6 (0.5)	15, (1.7%)	1, (6.7%)	1	879	0.85 (0.6)	4, (0.5%)	0, (0%)
2	874	3.4 (1.2)	33, (3.8%)	6, (18.2%)	2	873	4.4 (1.6)	27, (3.1%)	6, (22.2%)
3	876	9.5 (2.4)	47, (5.4%)	19, (40.4%)	3	876	12.2 (3.1)	49, (5.6%)	18, (36.7%)
4	876	21.5 (5.1)	68, (7.8%)	37, (54.4%)	4	876	40.9 (29.3)	83, (9.5%)	39, (47.0%)
Sum	3504	8.8 (8.5)	163, (4.65%)	63, (38.7%)	Sum	3504	14.6 (21.6)	163, (4.65%)	63, (38.7%)

In the same table, we show the percentage of mortality in the different quartiles of the second CRP test that was taken within 24 h from admission. Again, the seven day mortality rates increased according to the CRP increment being 0.5% in the first quartile as opposed to 9.5% in the fourth one (chi-square statistics was 85.0, $p < 0.0001$).

Therefore, while the death percentage was 4.6 times higher in the fourth as opposed to the first quartile of the first CRP test, this difference was 19 times higher in the fourth as opposed to the first quartile of the follow-up CRP test (second CRP measurement, right side of Table 1).

The lowest mortality rate was found in patients with the second measurement of CRP in the first quartile. These patients who arrived with a CRP below 31.9 mg/L and whose CRP concentrations remained minimal on the second day had a 3.4 times less mortality rate. Patients in the first CRP quartile of the first measurement presented a 0.5% mortality rate. Distinctly different, patients in the first CRP quartile of the first measurement demonstrated a 1.7% mortality percentage.

The negative predictive value of patients admitting to the Department of Internal Medicine with the first CRP <31.9 and second measurement of CRP in the lowest quartile (CRP <2 mg/L) was 0.0046.

The area under the ROC curve (AUC) when using the first CRP measurement as the predictor of 7 day mortality was 0.639 (0.599–0.680) $p < 0.001$. This AUC increased to 0.731 (0.696–0.766) $p < 0.001$ when using the second measurement of CRP.

Furthermore, the Cox regression using age, gender, and the first and second CRP quartiles together confirmed that the age and quartile of the second CRP measurements had a significant effect on mortality (hazard ratios (exp(b) being 1.08 for age, and 5.8, 10.0, and 14.1 for quartiles 2, 3, and 4, respectively, of the follow-up CRP test ($p \leq 0.001$ for all))) (Figure 1).

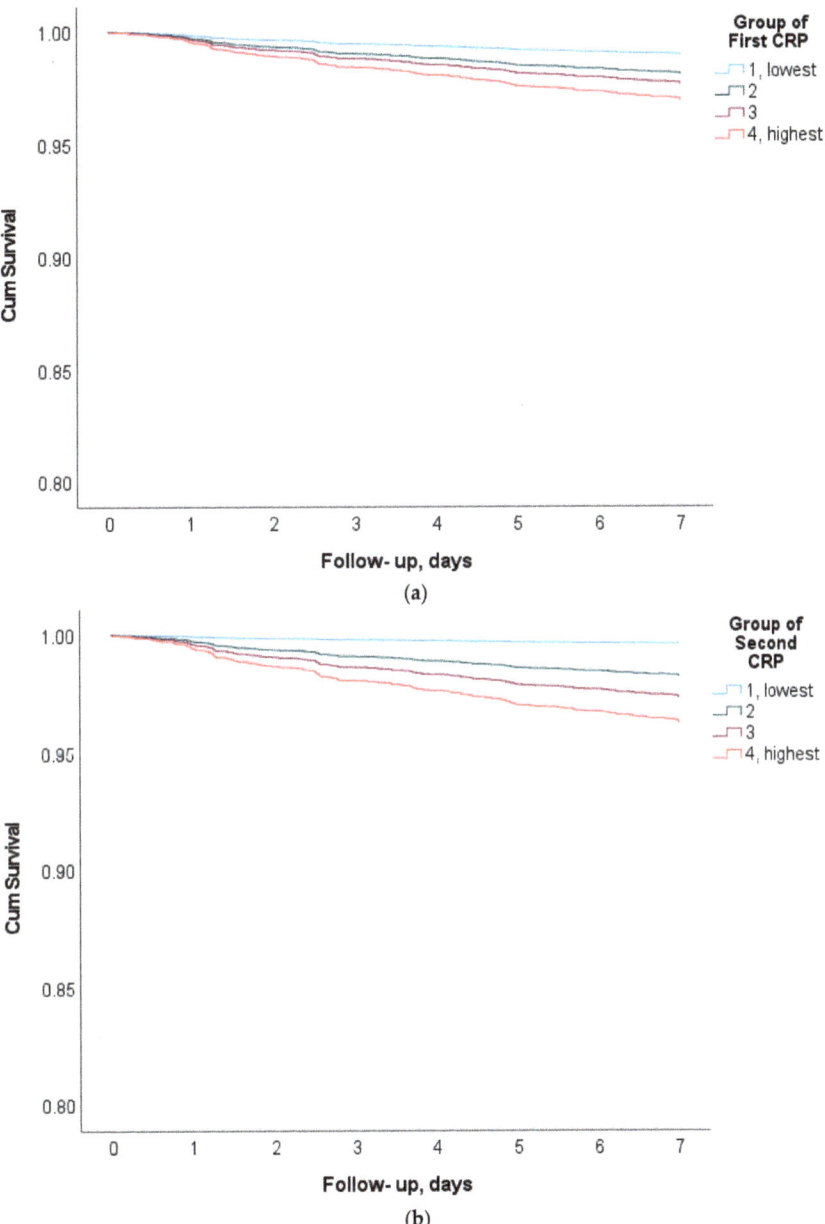

Figure 1. The survival plots for the first (**a**) and second (**b**) CRP quartiles (one is the lowest quartile, four is the highest). Log-rank mantel-Cox) < 0.001 for both.

Of special interest is our finding that the sepsis cause of deaths increased in a dose dependent manner with the quartiles of the first and second CRP. Patients with an extreme low level of CRP (first quartile) not only had aa better survival rate, but also had a lower risk of mortality from sepsis compared to patients at the highest quartile of either the first or second measurement of CRP (6.7% and 0% of mortality from sepsis for patients at the first quartile compared to 54.4% and 47.0% at the fourth quartile of the first and second CRP measurements, Table 3).

4. Discussion

To the best of our knowledge, this is the first study to explore the causes of death in patients who were admitted to the Department of Internal Medicine with apparently normal CRP concentration and in whom a follow-up CRP test was obtained within 24 h from admission. It was found, indeed, that despite presenting with a relatively low-grade inflammatory response that could potentially be observed in an apparently healthy population, these individuals might harbor severe and potentially lethal medical conditions. This concept was recently described by our group in patients who were admitted to the hospital with CRP concentrations that were below the detection level of the wr-CRP test [3].

We focused on the reasons of death in patients who were admitted to the Department of Internal Medicine with apparently normal CRP concentration and presented various degrees of inflammatory bursts by performing a follow-up CRP test within the first 24 h of their hospitalization. This study is especially relevant since it is known that the inflammatory response is not only a marker for the severity of the disease, but is involved in pathophysiological changes that could have deleterious effects, especially if exaggerated. This has clearly been shown in several clinical models such as in patients with ST-elevation myocardial infarction (STEMI) [16–18] as well as in the recent COVID-19 pandemic [19–21]. What we found is a gradual correlation between the intensity of the inflammatory response and the probability of death from different medical conditions within a relatively short period. These findings highly suggest not relying on a single apparently normal C-reactive protein CRP concentration upon admission to a medical facility, but insisting on at least one, if not more than one, additional test to follow.

The notion that the inflammatory response is a dynamic one and that the acute phase response has a well-established course is well-known [22]. However, due to economical availability as well as organizational difficulties, clinicians often do not perform repeated tests, and this is especially true in conditions where the results of the CRP test are not high. In fact, facing an individual with high CRP concentrations presents no special dilemmas to the clinician with regard to the question oof whether the patient has a significant inflammatory response or not. The main problem concentrates around those who seek medical care and do not present a heightened inflammatory response.

Although this article focused on CRP, it is important to mention that other markers could be used by clinicians to evaluate an inflammatory process such as hemoglobin, white blood cell count, fibrinogen, cytokines, chemokines, complement factors, adhesion molecules, and the blood sedimentation rate [23–28].With the advanced data-driven machine learning methods, we assumed that in the near future, it would be possible to handle multiple biomarkers simultaneously to gain a much more accurate mortality prediction [29–31].

There is no agreement in the medical literature or between researchers of what an apparently normal CRP concentration means. In an apparently healthy population, low risk for cardiovascular disease is defined as CRP <1 mg/L and high risk as >3 mg/L [32]. In order to cover the vast majority of apparently healthy individuals, we chose the cutoff of mean CRP plus three standard deviations, which was equal to 31.9 mg/L in our cohort of apparently healthy individuals who attended a routine annual health-screening program and had no signs or symptoms of an active inflammatory disease including specific questions that were asked regarding such an eventual active inflammatory disease/disorder. The details of this cohort have been extensively described in the past [11–14]. We then decided arbitrarily to define the apparently normal C-reactive protein CRP concentration as values that were below this upper + three standard deviations, although one could argue that this is too a high level. Nevertheless, we made this decision to cover almost all CRP concentrations that can be detected in a population that does not seek medical assistance for an acute illness.

Of special interest was the finding that the correlation between the intensity of the inflammatory burst and the seven day mortality was not limited to infectious conditions but included different acute medical conditions including stroke, respiratory failure, sudden cardiac arrest, and others (see Supplementary Table S1). In fact, inflammation-related clinical deterioration has been described in diseases and disorders that are not caused by infective organisms [33–36]. In addition, we showed that the lack of a follow-up inflammatory burst is associated with significantly less mortality. Although one may assume that the lack or minimal inflammatory burst is only a reflection of a less severe disease/disorder, looking at the evolution of the anti-inflammatory treatments given in the COVID-19 pandemic, we could also raise the possibility that the limited inflammatory burst contributed to a better prognosis. In fact, the inflammatory burst is not necessarily an innocent bystander, and early anti-inflammatory interventions could have a beneficial role in the evolution of the disease.

Finally, we draw attention to the fact that sepsis was the leading reason for seven day mortality in this cohort. This is especially relevant for daily practice, since we included a cohort of all comers and not necessarily those with infectious diseases. Although this observation should be further investigated, the appearance of a significant inflammatory burst in the Department of Internal Medicine should raise the possibility of an ongoing acute infection.

Some limitations of this study should be taken into consideration. The main limitation was that this was a retrospective observational study. In addition, sorting out a certain group of patients that have doubtful criteria for sepsis diagnosis and CRP below a certain threshold might impose a selection bias. However, all patients who met the inclusion criteria were admitted to the hospital in the context of suspicious clinical images, regardless of their CRP values, and all CRP measurements were conducted in a single lab using the same laboratory method. In addition, some possible confounders of CRP levels were not recorded in our database such as race. In our subsequent studies, we wish to evaluate these prospectively. Another limitation was the possibility of losing the significance of the association between the CRP values and the mortality rates due to other confounders in the regression model.

We can conclude that the appearance of a significant inflammatory burst in patients who are admitted to the Department of Internal Medicine is associated with a worse prognosis, and the possible existence of an ongoing acute infection should be taken into consideration. A first apparently normal CRP concentration should be followed by additional tests to exclude serious medical conditions with poor prognosis. Clinicians should not make any firm prognostic conclusions before additional tests are performed in these special populations.

Supplementary Materials: The following supporting information can be downloaded at: https://www.mdpi.com/article/10.3390/jcm11113151/s1, Table S1: Cause of death by quartiles of 1st and 2nd CRP measurements.

Author Contributions: Conceptualization, R.M., S.B., S.S.-T. and A.W.; Data curation, R.M., A.M., S.B. and S.S.-T.; Formal analysis, R.M., S.B. and S.S.-T.; Funding acquisition, I.S.; Investigation, R.M., A.M., S.B. and S.S.-T.; Methodology, S.B., O.R., I.G. and S.S.-T.; Project administration, S.B.; Resources, A.M., I.G. and S.S.-T.; Supervision, S.B., I.S. and O.R.; Validation, S.B., S.S.-T. and A.W.; Visualization, R.M. and S.S.-T.; Writing—original draft, R.M., H.B.-A. and S.B.; Writing—review & editing, R.M., H.B.-A., A.M., S.B., D.Z., I.S., O.R., S.S.-T. and A.W. All authors have read and agreed to the published version of the manuscript.

Funding: This work was supported in part by the Dalia and Arie Prashkovsky grant for biomedical research TLV2021-345.

Institutional Review Board System: The study was conducted according to the guidelines of the Declaration of Helsinki and approved by the Institutional Review Board of The Tel-Aviv Sourasky Medical Center (protocol code: 0491-17-TLV; date of approval: 7 November 2017).

Informed Consent Statement: Informed consent was not necessary due to the anonymity of the data used and this study being a retrospective medical record analysis.

Data Availability Statement: Data will be made available upon reasonable request.

Conflicts of Interest: The authors declare no conflict of interest.

References

1. Medzhitov, R. Origin and Physiological Roles of Inflammation. *Nature* **2008**, *454*, 428–435. [CrossRef] [PubMed]
2. Ahmed, A.U. An Overview of Inflammation: Mechanism and Consequences. *Front. Biol. China* **2011**, *6*, 274. [CrossRef]
3. Feigin, E.; Levinson, T.; Berliner, S.; Zeltser, D.; Itzhak, S.; Shenhar-Tsarfaty, S.; Egoz, E.; Meilik, A.; Goldiner, I.; Rogowski, O.; et al. Patients Who Are Admitted to the Department of Internal Medicine with a Very Low C-Reactive Protein Concentration. *Eur. J. Inflamm.* **2021**, *19*, 1–7. [CrossRef]
4. Goldberg, I.; Shalmon, D.; Shteinvil, R.; Berliner, S.; Paran, Y.; Zeltser, D.; Shapira, I.; Shenhar-Tsarfaty, S.; Meilik, A.; Wasserman, A.; et al. A Second C-Reactive Protein (CRP) Test to Detect Inflammatory Burst in Patients with Acute Bacterial Infections Presenting with a First Relatively Low CRP. *Medicine* **2020**, *99*, e22551. [CrossRef]
5. Bower, J.K.; Lazo, M.; Juraschek, S.P.; Selvin, E. Within-Person Variability in High-Sensitivity C-Reactive Protein. *Arch. Intern. Med.* **2012**, *172*, 1519–1521. [CrossRef] [PubMed]
6. Rocco, A.; Ringleb, P.A.; Grittner, U.; Nolte, C.H.; Schneider, A.; Nagel, S. Follow-up C-Reactive Protein Level Is More Strongly Associated with Outcome in Stroke Patients than Admission Levels. *Neurol. Sci.* **2015**, *36*, 2235–2241. [CrossRef]
7. Lee, J.H.; Lee, Y.H.; Park, Y.H.; Kim, Y.H.; Hong, C.K.; Cho, K.W.; Hwang, S.Y. The Difference in C-Reactive Protein Value between Initial and 24 Hours Follow-up (D-CRP) Data as a Predictor of Mortality in Organophosphate Poisoned Patients. *Clin. Toxicol.* **2013**, *51*, 29–34. [CrossRef]
8. Gill, D.; Sivakumaran, P.; Wilding, P.; Love, M.; Veltkamp, R.; Kar, A. Trends in C-Reactive Protein Levels Are Associated with Neurological Change Twenty-Four Hours after Thrombolysis for Acute Ischemic Stroke. *J. Stroke Cerebrovasc. Dis.* **2016**, *25*, 1966–1969. [CrossRef]
9. Levinson, T.; Tamir, N.; Shenhar-Tsarfaty, S.; Paran, Y.; Zeltser, D.; Shapira, I.; Halpern, P.; Meilik, A.; Raykhshtat, E.; Goldiner, I.; et al. The Potential Benefit of a Second C-Reactive Protein Measurement in Patients with Gram-Negative Bacteraemia Presenting to the Emergency Medicine Department. *Biomarkers* **2020**, *25*, 533–538. [CrossRef]
10. Wasserman, A.; Karov, R.; Shenhar-Tsarfaty, S.; Paran, Y.; Zeltser, D.; Shapira, I.; Trotzky, D.; Halpern, P.; Meilik, A.; Raykhshtat, E.; et al. Septic Patients Presenting with Apparently Normal C-Reactive Protein: A Point of Caution for the ER Physician. *Medicine* **2019**, *98*, e13989. [CrossRef]
11. Rogowski, O.; Toker, S.; Shapira, I.; Melamed, S.; Shirom, A.; Zeltser, D.; Berliner, S. Values of High-Sensitivity C-Reactive Protein in Each Month of the Year in Apparently Healthy Individuals. *Am. J. Cardiol.* **2005**, *95*, 152–155. [CrossRef] [PubMed]
12. Rogowski, O.; Shapira, I.; Peretz, H.; Berliner, S. Glycohaemoglobin as a Determinant of Increased Fibrinogen Concentrations and Low-Grade Inflammation in Apparently Healthy Nondiabetic Individuals. *Clin. Endocrinol.* **2008**, *68*, 182–189. [CrossRef] [PubMed]
13. Rogowski, O.; Shapira, I.; Bassat, O.K.-B.; Chundadze, T.; Finn, T.; Berliner, S.; Steinvil, A. Waist Circumference as the Predominant Contributor to the Micro-Inflammatory Response in the Metabolic Syndrome: A Cross Sectional Study. *J. Inflamm.* **2010**, *7*, 35. [CrossRef] [PubMed]
14. Ehrenwald, M.; Wasserman, A.; Shenhar-Tsarfaty, S.; Zeltser, D.; Friedensohn, L.; Shapira, I.; Berliner, S.; Rogowski, O. Exercise Capacity and Body Mass Index-Important Predictors of Change in Resting Heart Rate. *BMC Cardiovasc. Disord.* **2019**, *19*, 307–308. [CrossRef]
15. Rogowski, O.; Vered, Y.; Shapira, I.; Hirsh, M.; Zakut, V.; Berliner, S. Introducing the Wide Range C-Reactive Protein (Wr-CRP) into Clinical Use for the Detection of Microinflammation. *Clin. Chim. Acta* **2005**, *358*, 151–158. [CrossRef]
16. Holzknecht, M.; Tiller, C.; Reindl, M.; Lechner, I.; Fink, P.; Lunger, P.; Mayr, A.; Henninger, B.; Brenner, C.; Klug, G.; et al. Association of c-reactive protein velocity with early left ventricular dysfunction in patients with first st-elevation myocardial infarction. *J. Clin. Med.* **2021**, *10*, 5494. [CrossRef]
17. Banai, A.; Levit, D.; Morgan, S.; Loewenstein, I.; Merdler, I.; Hochstadt, A.; Szekely, Y.; Topilsky, Y.; Banai, S.; Shacham, Y. Association between C-Reactive Protein Velocity and Left Ventricular Function in Patients with ST-Elevated Myocardial Infarction. *J. Clin. Med.* **2022**, *11*, 401. [CrossRef]
18. Ries, W.; Torzewski, J.; Heigl, F.; Pfluecke, C.; Kelle, S.; Darius, H.; Ince, H.; Mitzner, S.; Nordbeck, P.; Butter, C.; et al. C-Reactive Protein Apheresis as Anti-inflammatory Therapy in Acute Myocardial Infarction: Results of the CAMI-1 Study. *Front. Cardiovasc. Med.* **2021**, *8*, 591714. [CrossRef]
19. Paces, J.; Strizova, Z.; Smrz, D.; Cerny, J. COVID-19 and the Immune System. *Physiol. Res.* **2020**, *69*, 379–388. [CrossRef]
20. Lazzaroni, M.G.; Piantoni, S.; Masneri, S.; Garrafa, E.; Martini, G.; Tincani, A.; Andreoli, L.; Franceschini, F. Coagulation Dysfunction in COVID-19: The Interplay between Inflammation, Viral Infection and the Coagulation System. *Blood Rev.* **2021**, *46*, 100745. [CrossRef]
21. Choudhary, S.; Sharma, K.; Silakari, O. The Interplay between Inflammatory Pathways and COVID-19: A Critical Review on Pathogenesis and Therapeutic Options. *Microb. Pathog.* **2021**, *150*, 104673. [CrossRef]
22. Gabay, C.; Kushner, I. Acute-Phase Proteins and Other Systemic Responses to Inflammation. *N. Engl. J. Med.* **1999**, *340*, 448–454. [CrossRef] [PubMed]

23. Tripepi, G.; Mallamaci, F.; Zoccali, C. Inflammation Markers, Adhesion Molecules, and All-Cause and Cardiovascular Mortality in Patients with ESRD: Searching for the Best Risk Marker by Multivariate Modeling. *J. Am. Soc. Nephrol.* **2005**, *16*, S83–S88. [CrossRef]
24. Faix, J.D. Biomarkers of Sepsis. *Crit. Rev. Clin. Lab. Sci.* **2013**, *50*, 23–36. [CrossRef] [PubMed]
25. Germolec, D.R.; Shipkowski, K.A.; Frawley, R.P.; Evans, E. Markers of Inflammation. *Methods Mol. Biol.* **2018**, *1803*, 57–79. [CrossRef] [PubMed]
26. Grondman, I.; Pirvu, A.; Riza, A.; Ioana, M.; Netea, M.G. Biomarkers of Inflammation and the Etiology of Sepsis. *Biochem. Soc. Trans.* **2020**, *48*, 1–14. [CrossRef]
27. Luyendyk, J.P.; Schoenecker, J.G.; Flick, M.J. The Multifaceted Role of Fibrinogen in Tissue Injury and Inflammation. *Blood* **2019**, *133*, 511–520. [CrossRef]
28. Lapić, I.; Padoan, A.; Bozzato, D.; Plebani, M. Erythrocyte Sedimentation Rate and C-Reactive Protein in Acute Inflammation. *Am. J. Clin. Pathol.* **2020**, *153*, 14–29. [CrossRef]
29. Lien, F.; Wang, H.Y.; Lu, J.J.; Wen, Y.H.; Chiueh, T.S. Predicting 2-Day Mortality of Thrombocytopenic Patients Based on Clinical Laboratory Data Using Machine Learning. *Med. Care* **2021**, *59*, 245–250. [CrossRef]
30. Moor, M.; Rieck, B.; Horn, M.; Jutzeler, C.R.; Borgwardt, K. Early Prediction of Sepsis in the ICU Using Machine Learning: A Systematic Review. *Front. Med.* **2021**, *8*, 607952. [CrossRef]
31. Tseng, Y.J.; Wang, H.Y.; Lin, T.W.; Lu, J.J.; Hsieh, C.H.; Liao, C.T. Development of a Machine Learning Model for Survival Risk Stratification of Patients with Advanced Oral Cancer. *JAMA Netw. Open* **2020**, *3*, e2011768. [CrossRef] [PubMed]
32. Pearson, T.A.; Mensah, G.A.; Alexander, R.W.; Anderson, J.L.; Cannon, R.O.; Criqui, M.; Fadl, Y.Y.; Fortmann, S.P.; Hong, Y.; Myers, G.L.; et al. Markers of Inflammation and Cardiovascular Disease. *Circulation* **2003**, *107*, 499–511. [CrossRef] [PubMed]
33. Lenz, A.; Franklin, G.A.; Cheadle, W.G. Systemic Inflammation after Trauma. *Injury* **2007**, *38*, 1336–1345. [CrossRef] [PubMed]
34. Hietbrink, F.; Koenderman, L.; Rijkers, G.T.; Leenen, L.P.H. Trauma: The Role of the Innate Immune System. *World J. Emerg. Surg.* **2006**, *1*, 15. [CrossRef]
35. Helmy, A.; de Simoni, M.G.; Guilfoyle, M.R.; Carpenter, K.L.H.; Hutchinson, P.J. Cytokines and Innate Inflammation in the Pathogenesis of Human Traumatic Brain Injury. *Prog. Neurobiol.* **2011**, *95*, 352–372. [CrossRef]
36. Huber-Lang, M.; Lambris, J.D.; Ward, P.A. Innate Immune Responses to Trauma. *Nat. Immunol.* **2018**, *19*, 327–341. [CrossRef]

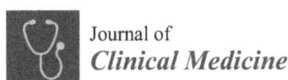

Review

Targeting C-Reactive Protein by Selective Apheresis in Humans: Pros and Cons

Jan Torzewski [1], Patrizia Brunner [2], Wolfgang Ries [3], Christoph D. Garlichs [3], Stefan Kayser [2], Franz Heigl [4] and Ahmed Sheriff [2,5,*]

1. Cardiovascular Center Oberallgaeu-Kempten, Clinic Association Allgaeu, 87439 Kempten, Germany; jan.torzewski@klinikverbund-allgaeu.de
2. Pentracor GmbH, 16761 Hennigsdorf, Germany; brunner@pentracor.de (P.B.); kayser@pentracor.de (S.K.)
3. Medical Clinic, Diakonissenhospital Flensburg, 24939 Flensburg, Germany; rieswo@diako.de (W.R.); garlichsch@diako.de (C.D.G.)
4. Medical Care Center Kempten-Allgaeu, 87439 Kempten, Germany; heigl@mvz-kempten.de
5. Division of Gastroenterology, Infectiology and Rheumatology, Medical Department, Charité University Medicine, 12200 Berlin, Germany
* Correspondence: ahmed.sheriff@charite.de

Abstract: C-reactive protein (CRP), the prototype human acute phase protein, may be causally involved in various human diseases. As CRP appeared much earlier in evolution than antibodies and nonetheless partly utilizes the same biological structures, it is likely that CRP has been the first antibody-like molecule in the evolution of the immune system. Like antibodies, CRP may cause autoimmune reactions in a variety of human pathologies. Consequently, therapeutic targeting of CRP may be of utmost interest in human medicine. Over the past two decades, however, pharmacological targeting of CRP has turned out to be extremely difficult. Currently, the easiest, most effective and clinically safest method to target CRP in humans may be the specific extracorporeal removal of CRP by selective apheresis. The latter has recently shown promising therapeutic effects, especially in acute myocardial infarction and COVID-19 pneumonia. This review summarizes the pros and cons of applying this novel technology to patients suffering from various diseases, with a focus on its use in cardiovascular medicine.

Keywords: inflammation; cardiovascular; COVID-19; arteriosclerosis; ischemic stroke; therapeutic apheresis

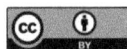

1. Introduction

In humans, C-reactive protein (CRP) activates the classical complement pathway via C1q [1] and stimulates macrophages via Fcγ-receptors [2,3]. Obviously, CRP utilizes the same biological structures as antibodies [4]. In further analogy, CRP may be causally involved in various human diseases by triggering (severe) ancient autoimmune reactions [5–7]. Although the latter hypothesis has been discussed in medical science since decades the issue has never been clarified. This is due to the fact that no drug or medical product targeting CRP has been on the market so far.

CRP synthesis and structure have extensively been reviewed elsewhere [8,9]. Here, we briefly review the role of CRP in physiology and pathophysiology with a focus on complement and macrophages. We then deal with the recent breakthrough in CRP targeting achieved by selective CRP apheresis. Pros and cons are listed in Table 1. Finally, we give an overview on current clinical trials and hypothesize on future developments. Thus, this review article may also be considered as an opinion paper.

Table 1. Pros and cons for CRP apheresis.

Pros	Cons
efficient and fast removal of large amounts of CRP within hours	blood plasma needs to be supplied to the adsorber instead of whole blood
regenerable immune adsorber→nearly unlimited capacity	the treatment takes approximately 5 h and needs to be repeated on successive days depending on the indication
approved by CE certification for removal of CRP	additional anticoagulation maybe critical in some patients
specific for CRP	(minimally) invasive procedure requiring peripheral venous access or Shaldon catheter
no removal of other molecules or medication	immunosuppression (?)
reusable adsorber	
apheresis is an established technique	

2. CRP in Physiology

CRP is expressed in the ancient Limulus for more than 250 million years ago [10]. Although evolutionarily highly conserved, there are significant species differences in CRP function [11]. In humans, CRP activates the classical complement pathway and opsonizes biological particles for macrophages via Fcγ-receptors [1–3,12]. The latter seems remarkable as these functions are also antibody functions: Thus, like CRP, antibodies activate the classical complement cascade and bind to Fcγ-receptors via their Fc-region [4]. CRP has appeared earlier in evolution than antibodies and may, consequently, be the first antibody analogue in the evolution of the immune system [13]. In ancient *Limulus*, which survives without the benefits of adaptive immunity, CRP is vital for host defense against bacterial infection [10]. In humans, however, having developed highly sophisticated adaptive immunity, CRP may rather be a relic of evolution and emerged to have a role in tissue regeneration [6]. When apoptotic or dying cells display lysophosphatidylcholine (oxidized phosphatidylcholine) in their membranes, CRP recognizes these cells and opsonizes them for Fcγ-receptor mediated removal by macrophages [14]. Thus, in human physiology, CRP may, above all, play a major role in the process of wound healing and removal of apoptotic and necrotic cells.

CRP is probably the most commonly measured inflammatory molecule in clinical medicine. Again, as CRP activates complement via C1q and stimulates macrophages via Fcγ-receptors (in analogy to antibodies) CRP may be considered as an early primitive antibody and a pathogenic factor rather than an inflammation marker only.

3. CRP in Pathophysiology

In pathophysiology, an active contribution of CRP to initiation and progression of disease has been discussed for decades [13,15,16]. This discussion has never come to an end because a definitive proof of CRP's causal involvement in disease in humans was lacking. Whereas the molecule's role as a marker of activity of infectious, autoimmune, ischemic or even cardiovascular disease [17] is well established and generally accepted, it is important to note that there is no international consensus on causal contribution of CRP to the pathogenesis of any human disease. In cardiovascular disease, mendelian randomization trials strongly contradict causality and active contribution of CRP to pathogenesis [18–20]. This is crucial. It is, however, also crucial to realize that Mendelian randomization has to be interpreted with care and is, by far, less reliable than randomization in clinical trials. The latter has been reviewed in detail in a number of noteworthy articles [21–24]. Regulation of CRP synthesis includes not only one but a number of genes [25–27] and thus, a one gene/one protein genetic approach might be problematic. In addition, the issue of canalization could be relevant in a protein that is as highly conserved as CRP. Finally, cardiovascular disease is complex and each disease entity deserves detailed analysis [13]. In particular, the pathophysiological role of CRP in acute events must be considered separately from that in chronic events. The evidence in the acute setting is overwhelming (please see Section 3.3.2), whereas the evidence in the chronic inflammatory setting is still being collected. Ultimately, randomized trials might clarify these issues much better than Mendelian randomization [28]. Randomized controlled trials, however, are only possible with an available specific and efficient therapy comparing treatment group to control group. Such therapy has only very recently become reality.

3.1. CRP in Viral and Bacterial Infection

CRP is one of the most frequently determined molecules in clinical medicine. In daily practice, it is used for the non-specific initial diagnosis of viral or bacterial infection and also for monitoring the course of such infection under medical therapy [29]. Especially, the success of antibiotic therapy in bacterial infection and sepsis is usually determined by measuring CRP levels in addition to clinical evaluation. Importantly, CRP plasma levels in viral infection are usually significantly lower than CRP levels in bacterial infection [30]. This is of particular importance when looking at COVID-19 disease (please see Section 3.5). Although COVID-19 patients suffer from a viral disease, CRP levels in COVID-19 patients with a bad prognosis are surprisingly high. Plasma levels up to 400 mg/L, usually seen in severe bacterial infection or sepsis only, are common in deleterious COVID pneumonia without superinfection [31].

3.2. CRP in Autoimmune Disease

Although the association between CRP and the activity of autoimmune disease is well known and highly suggestive for a causal involvement in this heterogeneous group of diseases (like rheumatoid arthritis, ulcerative colitis, Crohn's disease, psoriasis, giant cell arteritis etc.) [30], there are no studies on specific CRP inhibition in autoimmune disease. Notably, upstream interleukin-6 (IL-6) targeting with tocilizumab seems partly effective [32].

3.3. CRP in Cardiovascular Disease

3.3.1. Atherosclerosis

CRP plasma levels correlate with cardiovascular risk [17]. CRP accumulates in human atherosclerotic lesions [33] and exerts pro-atherogenic effects in vitro [13]. Some of the effects reported in the literature, especially on endothelial cells and vascular smooth muscle cells, however, have been shown to be caused by contamination of the used CRP preparations by either azide or lipopolysaccharide [34,35]. The latter seems reasonable as CRP interaction with ancient immune cells, i.e., macrophages, is visible in tissue specimen and seems more relevant than interaction with cells not contributing to the immune response. Mendelian trials, in awareness of their limitations, contradict the significant causal contribution of CRP to atherogenesis and its sequelae [18–20]. In contrast, recent large clinical trials suggest that the IL-1β/IL-6/CRP pathway is intimately involved in cardiovascular disease [36–38]. Specific and direct targeting of the CRP molecule, however, has never been tried yet. The only reason for this is the fact that, in spite of huge pharmacological effort, no CRP specific chemical inhibitor or antagonist has been available.

3.3.2. CRP in Myocardial Infarction

Acute myocardial infarction (AMI) implies a huge burden for the health system, since patients who recover still suffer from reduced quality of life and a high risk of severe complications later on. The risk correlates significantly with the extent of myocardial injury [39]. Especially innate immunity aggravates and extends myocardial injury [40,41]. Serum CRP concentrations during and after AMI correlate with clinical outcome and with larger infarct size [42–45]. This has been described for more than two decades now and is in line with the known pathological function of CRP: eliminating cells in the area at risk [6,46,47]. This area contains cells, which could recover after revascularization and reperfusion, but are sequentially destroyed by immune-mediated mechanisms. Numerous experimental approaches focusing specifically on AMI have shown this in detail [48–53]. Recently, it has been shown in the C-reactive protein apheresis in Acute Myocardial Infarction-1 (CAMI-1) study that the magnitude of infarct damage or reduction in cardiac output is significantly related to the amount of CRP synthesized by the patient immediately after the onset of his AMI. In the same study, significant evidence was also found that reduction in CRP levels conferred a better outcome in terms of infarct size and cardiac output. Some patients in the verum group (CRP apheresis group) even showed no scar at all (as assessed by cardiovascular magnetic resonance). These were not aborted infarctions, because aborted infarctions were treated as dropouts [5].

3.3.3. CRP in Myocarditis and Dilated Cardiomyopathy

In myocarditis, most frequently caused by viral infection [54], elevated CRP levels are common. Autoimmune myocarditis is also associated with high CRP plasma levels. Chronic myocarditis is known to trigger the development of dilated cardiomyopathy [54], a disease leading to ongoing heart failure not only in elder but also in younger patients. It is noteworthy that CRP and complement deposits have been shown to be frequently present in myocardial biopsy specimen obtained from patients suffering from dilated cardiomyopathy [55].

3.4. CRP in Neurological Disorders and Stroke

Ischemic stroke exhibits similar pathological mechanisms to AMI. To date, restoring rapid reperfusion of the brain constitutes the only established therapeutic strategy to reduce the size of the infarct and the consequences of the disease [56]. However, inflammation plays an important role in various stages of ischemic stroke. Several humoral and cellular mechanisms are set in motion by the occlusion and subsequent therapeutic reperfusion [57]. Several findings substantiate the hypothesis that CRP plays an identical pathological role as shown in AMI, facilitating the elimination of energetically challenged and compromised cells in the penumbra.

The early inflammatory response after stroke has been identified as a key prognostic factor [58,59]. Patients with favorable clinical outcome feature significantly lower levels of inflammatory parameters, especially CRP, compared to patients with poor outcome [60–62]. Muir et al. have shown that CRP levels measured within 72 h after stroke predict mortality over an observation period of up to 4 years [63]. Further, studies in a rat animal model have shown that infusion of human CRP enlarges cerebral infarct areas after acute occlusion via a complement-dependent mechanism [64].

3.5. CRP in COVID-19

COVID-19 is a virus-induced disease, but it also includes an important immune and autoimmune component. CRP was used early on during the pandemic as a marker for the severity and progression of the disease in patients, as it increases dramatically together with IL-6 during the clinical manifestation of COVID-19 [65–68]. The validity of CRP as a significant predictor of the outcome in COVID-19 was confirmed many times. A rapid increase in CRP allows the prognosis of ventilatory requirement of patients as well as their clinical outcome [31]. CRP levels further correlate with computed tomography (CT) findings in COVID-19 patients [69].

Corresponding to these findings, abundant amounts of CRP and complement deposits and were found in the lungs of deceased COVID-19 patients, including mainly C1q [70,71].

Severe progression occurs in roughly 14% of patients suffering from COVID-19 and in 5% this can lead to ventilator dependency with a serious prognosis [68,72–74]. An important therapeutic approach focuses on the treatment of acute respiratory failure—a major cause of mortality, followed by cardiac and septic complications. In the severe course of the disease, there is an initial cytokine storm, accompanied by a massive increase in the CRP concentration, followed by pulmonary fibrosis [75,76].

Intra-alveolar edema and hemorrhage are common observations in the lungs of COVID-19 patients, resulting in ischemic alveolar tissue. In COVID-19 pneumonia, there is massive damage to the alveoli as well as thrombus formation in the microcirculation. Complement binding to CRP leads to immigration of macrophages and, via increased expression of tissue factor, to thrombus formation. Both are exacerbated by high CRP levels and parallel to the underlying pathomechanism in other diseases, CRP causally enlarges destroyed tissue and contributes to irreversible tissue destruction [77].

These findings support the hypothesis stated early on that targeting CRP therapeutically can inhibit the lung deterioration and disease progression [6,7,78,79]. This innovative therapeutic approach for the early phase of severe COVID-19 is currently being used in three German hospitals. Three of the treated cases and one case series have already been published [7,80–82] and another publication on a case series has been submitted and can be viewed as a preprint (https://www.preprints.org/manuscript/202203.0029/v1; 16 March 2022). In the case series by Esposito et al., there is a marked improvement in COVID-19 pneumonia on imaging performed before and after CRP apheresis.

4. Why May CRP Apheresis Be a Breakthrough in CRP Targeting?

Over more than two decades, several approaches to target CRP have been discussed and tried by various researchers and pharmaceutical companies. These approaches include:

- CRP inhibition by antisense technologies [83];
- CRP inhibition by small molecular weight inhibitors [84];
- Inhibition of hepatic CRP synthesis [85];
- Inhibition of CRP mediated complement activation;
- Inhibition of CRP binding to its receptors.

Each of these approaches was well justified and was also partly promising. Interestingly, however, none of them resulted in a specific substance or medication that was applicable in human clinical practice. The latter seems remarkable because all the people and companies involved were well experienced in drug development. Several reasons were causal for the problems in generating specific CRP inhibitors: Antisense technology was, up to present day, not sufficiently effective. Small molecular weight inhibitors have not yet been transferred to human application. For inhibition of hepatic CRP synthesis, no specific novel substance was identified. Blockage of CRP-mediated complement activation and its C1q binding site turned out to be difficult for steric reasons. Inhibition of CRP binding to its receptors was also impossible because CRP receptors are also antibody receptors and thus, this approach may result in severe immunosuppression. Generally spoken, CRP—in its pentameric structure—is a molecule with structural redundancies difficult to interfere with. Its synthesis is complexly regulated involving different gene loci and furthermore, its highly dynamic regulation involving an up to 10,000-fold increase in plasma levels within few hours during acute phase response counteract an efficient synthesis inhibition or targeting.

The most important clinical concern about CRP targeting is the danger of immunosuppression with consecutive bacterial or viral infection and sepsis. Interestingly, in spite of significant reduction of CRP plasma levels via CRP apheresis in both disease entities, we have not observed such effects in our patients suffering from acute myocardial infarction or COVID-19 disease [5,7,80–82]. Thus, either CRP is not crucial in immune defense against microbial pathogens or the remaining CRP plasma levels after CRP apheresis are still sufficient. CRP apheresis is highly specific and does not relevantly influence other inflammatory markers or medication [86]. In the clinical setting, the most relevant apheresis procedure is lipid apheresis which mainly targets lipids and is far less specific [87,88].

Very often in clinical medicine simple approaches have turned out to be the best ones. Consequently, the idea to selectively remove CRP from the human plasma by specific and highly efficient extracorporeal apheresis [52] lacking severe side effects may finally turn out to be superior to other approaches. CRP apheresis may become beneficial in clinical medicine. This potential benefit, however, needs to be proven and fostered by an additional clinical trial program. The latter is currently ongoing.

5. Clinical Trials

"First in man"-application of CRP apheresis has been published in 2018 for a ST elevation myocardial infarction (STEMI) patient [89]. In this patient, post STEMI CRP plasma levels were lowered effectively and the patient experienced no side effects from CRP apheresis. The same was published for a small cohort of STEMI patients in 2019 [90]. The first and also the only clinical study on CRP apheresis in STEMI patients published up to the present day is the C-reactive protein apheresis in Acute Myocardial Infarction-1 (CAMI-1) study [5]. CAMI-1 was a non-randomized multi-center pilot study which has investigated feasibility and safety of CRP apheresis. Although the clinical observations were promising and the significant correlation between post-infarction CRP amount and myocardial infarct size was significantly lost in the treatment group, CAMI-1 cannot be regarded as being conclusive because it was not randomized.

Clinical trials including apheresis present the issue of an adequate sham control and a double-blind design. Although a sham control is biostatistically speaking crucial in order to get valid results that are not biased by the placebo effect, including this in the apheresis procedure is ethically challenging. Few apheresis trials included adequate sham controls, one of the best examples being granulocyte/monocyte apheresis in chronic gut diseases [91,92]. Here, control patients were subjected to the same extracorporeal circuit, but blood was bypassed and did not pass the column. As patients and clinicians were blinded and only the conducting apheresis team knew which patients received the sham procedure these trials were considered double-blind. This could be a feasible design for future CRP apheresis trials. However, the underlying disease has to be taken into consideration. After STEMI, ischemic stroke and during COVID-19, patients are hospitalized and already in critical state. Submitting them to a 4–6 h extracorporeal circuit and sham procedure is ethically not justifiable. Hence, most apheresis trials do not include a sham control and have either historical controls or patients that receive standard therapy without apheresis [93].

Current clinical trials investigating the effect of CRP apheresis on the course of various human diseases are summarized on the Website of U.S. National Library of Medicine/ClinicalTrials.gov (https://www.clinicaltrials.gov/ct2/results?term=C-reactive+protein+apheresis, accessed on 16 March 2022).

Two of the studies attract special attention because, for their randomized, controlled, multi-center design, they can be considered as proof of principle trials. One of them is the "CRP Apheresis in STEMI"-trial (NCT04939805), initiated by University of Innsbruck, Austria, a randomized, multi-center interventional trial including 170 patients and comparing standard therapy of STEMI plus CRP apheresis to standard therapy alone. The study largely follows the CAMI-1 protocol, it is well-planned and well-organized. Whether it is adequately powered to finally detect statistically significant differences in a disease with heterogeneous underlying anatomy and pathology is a matter of concern. In this context, the CAMI-1 registry, a multi-center all-comer CRP apheresis in AMI registry may help to identify patient subgroups that profit best and may also help to plan another randomized trial with modified inclusion criteria.

The second study attracting special attention is the "CRP Apheresis for Attenuation of Pulmonary, Myocardial and/or Kidney Injury in COVID-19"-trial (NCT04898062), a randomized, controlled, multi-center interventional trial initiated by the University of Essen, Germany, including 50 patients and comparing standard therapy of COVID-19 plus CRP apheresis to standard therapy alone. This study is of considerable importance. It is based on the pathophysiological hypothesis that CRP, in COVID-19, triggers a fulminant innate immunity autoimmune reaction in the human body which may be the real cause for the deleterious course in subjects with severe COVID-19 (Please see Section 3.5). Like CAMI-1, it is based on published case reports and case series strongly suggesting that only few participants may power such a randomized study adequately in order to prove a therapeutic benefit of CRP apheresis in severe COVID-19 disease [7,80,82]. If so, this small trial might become a benchmark trial in demonstrating conclusively that CRP is a trigger of ischemia induced autoimmune responses in the human body.

Whether CRP apheresis is useful in atherosclerosis, myocarditis and dilated cardiomyopathy, neurological disorders and stroke, or even in autoimmune disease, requires further systematic investigation. As CRP apheresis is not yet a broadly established therapy, we propose to treat patients within a reputable scientific framework only, i.e., within a scientific registry or randomized, controlled trial.

6. Discussion and Future Developments

CRP has been the first antibody-like molecule in the evolution of the immune system. Surprisingly, although it appeared earlier in evolution than nowadays antibodies, CRP utilizes the same biological structures (C1q, FcγRs) and, by doing this, has similar functions as modern antibodies (activation of classical complement cascade, opsonization of biological particles for macrophages). Notably, like antibodies, CRP may cause autoimmune reactions in the human body. First, clinical evidence for this comes from a clinical pilot study on using C-reactive protein apheresis as an add on-treatment of myocardial infarction (CAMI-1) and from case reports on successful use of C-reactive protein apheresis in COVID-19 disease.

A definitive proof of principle, however, is still lacking, With the initiation of "CRP Apheresis in STEMI" and "CRP Apheresis for Attenuation of Pulmonary, Myocardial and/or Kidney Injury in COVID-19", two randomized multicenter trials on C-reactive protein apheresis in STEMI on the one hand and COVID-19 on the other hand, a big step forward is to be expected soon after completion. These randomized trials are flanked by a number of clinical registries that may help to identify patient subgroups that strongly benefit from CRP apheresis. Finally, patients suffering from other acute and chronic diseases, in which CRP levels inversely correlate with prognosis (f. e. stroke, ulcerative colitis, Crohn's disease, pancreatitis, chronic polyarthritis, atherosclerosis etc.) might benefit from CRP apheresis in the future.

Author Contributions: J.T., P.B. and A.S. wrote the first draft, conceptualized and finalized the manuscript. C.D.G., W.R., S.K. and F.H. made substantial corrections. All authors have read and agreed to the published version of the manuscript.

Funding: No funding was applied to writing this review.

Institutional Review Board Statement: Not applicable.

Informed Consent Statement: Not applicable.

Conflicts of Interest: Ahmed Sheriff is Founder and Shareholder of Pentracor GmbH. Patrizia Brunner and Stefan Kayser are employees of Pentracor GmbH.

References

1. Kaplan, M.H.; Volanakis, J.E. Interaction of C-reactive protein complexes with the complement system. I. Consumption of human complement associated with the reaction of C-reactive protein with pneumococcal C-polysaccharide and with the choline phosphatides, lecithin and sphingomyelin. *J. Immunol.* **1974**, *112*, 2135–2147. [PubMed]
2. Bharadwaj, D.; Stein, M.P.; Volzer, M.; Mold, C.; Du Clos, T.W. The major receptor for C-reactive protein on leukocytes is fcgamma receptor II. *J. Exp. Med.* **1999**, *190*, 585–590. [CrossRef] [PubMed]
3. Manolov, D.E.; Röcker, C.; Hombach, V.; Nienhaus, G.U.; Torzewski, J. Ultrasensitive Confocal Fluorescence Microscopy of C-Reactive Protein Interacting With FcγRIIa. *Arter. Thromb. Vasc. Biol.* **2004**, *24*, 2372–2377. [CrossRef] [PubMed]
4. Daëron, M. Fc Receptor Biology. *Annu. Rev. Immunol.* **1997**, *15*, 203–234. [CrossRef]
5. Ries, W.; Torzewski, J.; Heigl, F.; Pfluecke, C.; Kelle, S.; Darius, H.; Ince, H.; Mitzner, S.; Nordbeck, P.; Butter, C.; et al. C-Reactive Protein Apheresis as Anti-inflammatory Therapy in Acute Myocardial Infarction: Results of the CAMI-1 Study. *Front. Cardiovasc. Med.* **2021**, *8*, 591714. [CrossRef]
6. Sheriff, A.; Kayser, S.; Brunner, P.; Vogt, B. C-Reactive Protein Triggers Cell Death in Ischemic Cells. *Front. Immunol.* **2021**, *12*, 630430. [CrossRef]

7. Torzewski, J.; Heigl, F.; Zimmermann, O.; Wagner, F.; Schumann, C.; Hettich, R.; Bock, C.; Kayser, S.; Sheriff, A. First-in-Man: Case Report of Selective C-Reactive Protein Apheresis in a Patient with SARS-CoV-2 Infection. *Am. J. Case Rep.* **2020**, *21*, e925020. [CrossRef]
8. Pepys, M.B.; Hirschfield, G. C-reactive protein: A critical update. *J. Clin. Investig.* **2003**, *111*, 1805–1812. [CrossRef]
9. Szalai, A.J.; Agrawal, A.; Greenhough, T.J.; Volanakis, J.E. C-reactive protein: Structural biology, gene expression, and host defense function. *Immunol. Res.* **1997**, *16*, 127–136. [CrossRef]
10. Nguyen, N.Y.; Suzuki, A.; Cheng, S.M.; Zon, G.; Liu, T.Y. Isolation and characterization of Limulus C-reactive protein genes. *J. Biol. Chem.* **1986**, *261*, 10450–10455. [CrossRef]
11. Torzewski, M.; Waqar, A.B.; Fan, J. Animal Models of C-Reactive Protein. *Mediat. Inflamm.* **2014**, *2014*, 683598. [CrossRef] [PubMed]
12. Mortensen, R.F.; Osmand, A.P.; Lint, T.F.; Gewurz, H. Interaction of C-reactive protein with lymphocytes and monocytes: Complement-dependent adherence and phagocytosis. *J. Immunol.* **1976**, *117*, 774–781. [PubMed]
13. Zimmermann, O.; Li, K.; Zaczkiewicz, M.; Graf, M.; Liu, Z.; Torzewski, J. C-Reactive Protein in Human Atherogenesis: Facts and Fiction. *Mediat. Inflamm.* **2014**, *2014*, 561428. [CrossRef] [PubMed]
14. Sproston, N.R.; Ashworth, J.J. Role of C-Reactive Protein at Sites of Inflammation and Infection. *Front. Immunol.* **2018**, *9*, 754. [CrossRef]
15. Pepys, M.B. C-reactive protein is neither a marker nor a mediator of atherosclerosis. *Nat. Clin. Pract. Nephrol.* **2008**, *4*, 234–235. [CrossRef]
16. Schunkert, H.; Samani, N.J. Elevated C-Reactive Protein in Atherosclerosis—Chicken or Egg? *N. Engl. J. Med.* **2008**, *359*, 1953–1955. [CrossRef]
17. Pearson, T.A.; Mensah, G.A.; Alexander, R.W.; Anderson, J.L.; Cannon, R.O., III; Criqui, M.; Fadl, Y.Y.; Fortmann, S.P.; Hong, Y.; Myers, G.L.; et al. Markers of Inflammation and Cardiovascular Disease: Application to Clinical and Public Health Practice: A Statement for Healthcare Professionals from the Centers for Disease Control and Prevention and the American Heart Association. *Circulation* **2003**, *107*, 499–511. [CrossRef]
18. Wensley, F.; Gao, P.; Burgess, S.; Kaptoge, S.; di Angelantonio, E.; Shah, T.; Engert, J.C.; Clarke, R.; Davey-Smith, G.; Nordestgaard, B.G.; et al. Association between C reactive protein and coronary heart disease: Mendelian randomisation analysis based on individual participant data. *BMJ* **2011**, *342*, d548. [CrossRef]
19. Elliott, P.; Chambers, J.C.; Zhang, W.; Clarke, R.; Hopewell, J.C.; Peden, J.F.; Erdmann, J.; Braund, P.; Engert, J.C.; Bennett, D.; et al. Genetic Loci Associated With C-Reactive Protein Levels and Risk of Coronary Heart Disease. *JAMA* **2009**, *302*, 37–48. [CrossRef]
20. Zacho, J.; Tybjaerg-Hansen, A.; Jensen, J.S.; Grande, P.; Sillesen, H.; Nordestgaard, B.G. Genetically Elevated C-Reactive Protein and Ischemic Vascular Disease. *N. Engl. J. Med.* **2008**, *359*, 1897–1908. [CrossRef]
21. Glynn, R.J. Promises and Limitations of Mendelian Randomization for Evaluation of Biomarkers. *Clin. Chem.* **2010**, *56*, 388–390. [CrossRef] [PubMed]
22. Morita, H.; Nagai, R. Genetically elevated C-reactive protein and vascular disease. *N. Engl. J. Med.* **2009**, *360*, 934, author reply 934–935. [PubMed]
23. Smith, G.D.; Ebrahim, S. "Mendelian randomization": Can genetic epidemiology contribute to understanding environmental determinants of disease? *Int. J. Epidemiol.* **2003**, *32*, 1–22. [CrossRef] [PubMed]
24. Smith, G.D.; Ebrahim, S. Mendelian randomization: Prospects, potentials, and limitations. *Int. J. Epidemiol.* **2004**, *33*, 30–42. [CrossRef] [PubMed]
25. Agrawal, A.; Cha-Molstad, H.; Samols, D.; Kushner, I. Transactivation of C-Reactive Protein by IL-6 Requires Synergistic Interaction of CCAAT/Enhancer Binding Protein β (C/EBPβ) and Rel p50. *J. Immunol.* **2001**, *166*, 2378–2384. [CrossRef] [PubMed]
26. Singh, P.P.; Voleti, B.; Agrawal, A. A Novel RBP-Jκ-Dependent Switch from C/EBPβ to C/EBPζ at the C/EBP Binding Site on the C-Reactive Protein Promoter. *J. Immunol.* **2007**, *178*, 7302–7309. [CrossRef]
27. Young, D.P.; Kushner, I.; Samols, D. Binding of C/EBPβ to the C-Reactive Protein (CRP) Promoter in Hep3B Cells Is Associated with Transcription of CRP mRNA. *J. Immunol.* **2008**, *181*, 2420–2427. [CrossRef]
28. Torzewski, J.; Fan, J.; Schunkert, H.; Szalai, A.J.; Torzewski, M. C-Reactive Protein and Arteriosclerosis. *Mediat. Inflamm.* **2014**, *2014*, 646817. [CrossRef]
29. Fernandez-Carballo, B.L.; Escadafal, C.; MacLean, E.; Kapasi, A.J.; Dittrich, S. Distinguishing bacterial versus non-bacterial causes of febrile illness—A systematic review of host biomarkers. *J. Infect.* **2021**, *82*, 1–10. [CrossRef]
30. Du Clos, T.W. C-reactive protein as a regulator of autoimmunity and inflammation. *Arthritis Care Res.* **2003**, *48*, 1475–1477. [CrossRef]
31. Smilowitz, N.R.; Kunichoff, D.; Garshick, M.; Shah, B.; Pillinger, M.; Hochman, J.S.; Berger, J.S. C-reactive protein and clinical outcomes in patients with COVID-19. *Eur. Heart J.* **2021**, *42*, 2270–2279. [CrossRef] [PubMed]
32. Serling-Boyd, N.; Wallace, Z.S. Management of primary vasculitides with biologic and novel small molecule medications. *Curr. Opin. Rheumatol.* **2020**, *33*, 8–14. [CrossRef]
33. Torzewski, J.; Torzewski, M.; Bowyer, D.E.; Fröhlich, M.; Koenig, W.; Waltenberger, J.; Fitzsimmons, C.; Hombach, V. C-Reactive Protein Frequently Colocalizes With the Terminal Complement Complex in the Intima of Early Atherosclerotic Lesions of Human Coronary Arteries. *Arter. Thromb. Vasc. Biol.* **1998**, *18*, 1386–1392. [CrossRef] [PubMed]

34. Berg, C.W.V.D.; Taylor, K.E.; Lang, D. C-Reactive Protein-Induced In Vitro Vasorelaxation Is an Artefact Caused by the Presence of Sodium Azide in Commercial Preparations. *Arter. Thromb. Vasc. Biol.* **2004**, *24*, e168–e171. [CrossRef]
35. Taylor, K.E.; Giddings, J.C.; Berg, C.W.V.D. C-Reactive Protein–Induced In Vitro Endothelial Cell Activation Is an Artefact Caused by Azide and Lipopolysaccharide. *Arter. Thromb. Vasc. Biol.* **2005**, *25*, 1225–1230. [CrossRef]
36. Ridker, P.M.; Danielson, E.; Fonseca, F.A.; Genest, J.; Gotto, A.M., Jr.; Kastelein, J.J.; Koenig, W.; Libby, P.; Lorenzatti, A.J.; MacFadyen, J.G.; et al. Rosuvastatin to Prevent Vascular Events in Men and Women with Elevated C-Reactive Protein. *N. Engl. J. Med.* **2008**, *359*, 2195–2207. [CrossRef]
37. Ridker, P.M.; Everett, B.M.; Thuren, T.; MacFadyen, J.G.; Chang, W.H.; Ballantyne, C.; Fonseca, F.; Nicolau, J.; Koenig, W.; Anker, S.D.; et al. Antiinflammatory Therapy with Canakinumab for Atherosclerotic Disease. *N. Engl. J. Med.* **2017**, *377*, 1119–1131. [CrossRef]
38. Tardif, J.-C.; Kouz, S.; Waters, D.D.; Bertrand, O.F.; Diaz, R.; Maggioni, A.P.; Pinto, F.J.; Ibrahim, R.; Gamra, H.; Kiwan, G.S.; et al. Efficacy and Safety of Low-Dose Colchicine after Myocardial Infarction. *N. Engl. J. Med.* **2019**, *381*, 2497–2505. [CrossRef]
39. De Waha, S.; Patel, M.R.; Granger, C.B.; Ohman, E.M.; Maehara, A.; Eitel, I.; Ben-Yehuda, O.; Jenkins, P.; Thiele, H.; Stone, G.W. Relationship between microvascular obstruction and adverse events following primary percutaneous coronary intervention for ST-segment elevation myocardial infarction: An individual patient data pooled analysis from seven randomized trials. *Eur. Heart J.* **2017**, *38*, 3502–3510. [CrossRef]
40. Frangogiannis, N.; Smith, C.; Entman, M.L. The inflammatory response in myocardial infarction. *Cardiovasc. Res.* **2002**, *53*, 31–47. [CrossRef]
41. Ong, S.-B.; Hernández-Reséndiz, S.; Crespo-Avilan, G.E.; Mukhametshina, R.T.; Kwek, X.-Y.; Cabrera-Fuentes, H.A.; Hausenloy, D.J. Inflammation following acute myocardial infarction: Multiple players, dynamic roles, and novel therapeutic opportunities. *Pharmacol. Ther.* **2018**, *186*, 73–87. [CrossRef] [PubMed]
42. Beranek, J.T. C-reactive protein and complement in myocardial infarction and postinfarction heart failure. *Eur. Heart J.* **1997**, *18*, 1834–1835. [CrossRef] [PubMed]
43. Liu, D.; Qi, X.; Li, Q.; Jia, W.; Wei, L.; Huang, A.; Liu, K.; Li, Z. Increased complements and high-sensitivity C-reactive protein predict heart failure in acute myocardial infarction. *Biomed. Rep.* **2016**, *5*, 761–765. [CrossRef] [PubMed]
44. Mani, P.; Puri, R.; Schwartz, G.G.; Nissen, S.E.; Shao, M.; Kastelein, J.J.P.; Menon, V.; Lincoff, A.M.; Nicholls, S. Association of Initial and Serial C-Reactive Protein Levels with Adverse Cardiovascular Events and Death after Acute Coronary Syndrome: A Secondary Analysis of the VISTA-16 Trial. *JAMA Cardiol.* **2019**, *4*, 314–320. [CrossRef]
45. Suleiman, M.; Khatib, R.; Agmon, Y.; Mahamid, R.; Boulos, M.; Kapeliovich, M.; Levy, Y.; Beyar, R.; Markiewicz, W.; Hammerman, H.; et al. Early Inflammation and Risk of Long-Term Development of Heart Failure and Mortality in Survivors of Acute Myocardial Infarction: Predictive Role of C-Reactive Protein. *J. Am. Coll. Cardiol.* **2006**, *47*, 962–968. [CrossRef]
46. Kayser, S.; Brunner, P.; Althaus, K.; Dorst, J.; Sheriff, A. Selective Apheresis of C-Reactive Protein for Treatment of Indications with Elevated CRP Concentrations. *J. Clin. Med.* **2020**, *9*, 2947. [CrossRef]
47. Kunze, R. C-Reactive Protein: From Biomarker to Trigger of Cell Death? *Ther. Apher. Dial.* **2019**, *23*, 494–496. [CrossRef]
48. Barrett, T.D.; Hennan, J.K.; Marks, R.M.; Lucchesi, B.R. C-Reactive-Protein-Associated Increase in Myocardial Infarct Size After Ischemia/Reperfusion. *J. Pharmacol. Exp. Ther.* **2002**, *303*, 1007–1013. [CrossRef]
49. Griselli, M.; Herbert, J.; Hutchinson, W.; Taylor, K.; Sohail, M.; Krausz, T.; Pepys, M. C-Reactive Protein and Complement Are Important Mediators of Tissue Damage in Acute Myocardial Infarction. *J. Exp. Med.* **1999**, *190*, 1733–1740. [CrossRef]
50. Lagrand, W.K.; Niessen, H.W.; Wolbink, G.-J.; Jaspars, L.H.; Visser, C.A.; Verheugt, F.W.; Meijer, C.J.; Hack, C.E. C-Reactive Protein Colocalizes With Complement in Human Hearts During Acute Myocardial Infarction. *Circulation* **1997**, *95*, 97–103. [CrossRef]
51. Nijmeijer, R.; Lagrand, W.K.; Lubbers, Y.T.; Visser, C.A.; Meijer, C.J.; Niessen, H.W.; Hack, C.E. C-Reactive Protein Activates Complement in Infarcted Human Myocardium. *Am. J. Pathol.* **2003**, *163*, 269–275. [CrossRef]
52. Sheriff, A.; Schindler, R.; Vogt, B.; Abdel-Aty, H.; Unger, J.K.; Bock, C.; Gebauer, F.; Slagman, A.; Jerichow, T.; Mans, D.; et al. Selective apheresis of C-reactive protein: A new therapeutic option in myocardial infarction? *J. Clin. Apher.* **2014**, *30*, 15–21. [CrossRef] [PubMed]
53. Valtchanova-Matchouganska, A.; Gondwe, M.; Nadar, A. The role of C-reactive protein in ischemia/reperfusion injury and preconditioning in a rat model of myocardial infarction. *Life Sci.* **2004**, *75*, 901–910. [CrossRef] [PubMed]
54. Tschöpe, C.; Ammirati, E.; Bozkurt, B.; Caforio, A.L.P.; Cooper, L.T.; Felix, S.B.; Hare, J.M.; Heidecker, B.; Heymans, S.; Hübner, N.; et al. Myocarditis and inflammatory cardiomyopathy: Current evidence and future directions. *Nat. Rev. Cardiol.* **2020**, *18*, 169–193. [CrossRef] [PubMed]
55. Zimmermann, O.; Bienek-Ziolkowski, M.; Wolf, B.; Vetter, M.; Baur, R.; Mailänder, V.; Hombach, V.; Torzewski, J. Myocardial inflammation and non-ischaemic heart failure: Is there a role for C-reactive protein? *Basic Res. Cardiol.* **2009**, *104*, 591–599. [CrossRef] [PubMed]
56. Catanese, L.; Tarsia, J.; Fisher, M. Acute Ischemic Stroke Therapy Overview. *Circ. Res.* **2017**, *120*, 541–558. [CrossRef] [PubMed]
57. Anrather, J.; Iadecola, C. Inflammation and Stroke: An Overview. *Neurotherapeutics* **2016**, *13*, 661–670. [CrossRef]
58. Montaner, J.; Fernandez-Cade, I.; Molina, C.A.; Ribo, M.; Huertas, R.; Rosell, A.; Penalba, A.; Ortega, L.; Chacón, P.; Alvarez-Sabin, J. Poststroke C-Reactive Protein Is a Powerful Prognostic Tool Among Candidates for Thrombolysis. *Stroke* **2006**, *37*, 1205–1210. [CrossRef]

59. Winbeck, K.; Poppert, H.; Etgen, T.; Conrad, B.; Sander, D. Prognostic Relevance of Early Serial C-Reactive Protein Measurements After First Ischemic Stroke. *Stroke* **2002**, *33*, 2459–2464. [CrossRef]
60. Di Napoli, M.; Papa, F.; Bocola, V. Prognostic Influence of Increased C-Reactive Protein and Fibrinogen Levels in Ischemic Stroke. *Stroke* **2001**, *32*, 133–138. [CrossRef]
61. Di Napoli, M.; Schwaninger, M.; Cappelli, R.; Ceccarelli, E.; Di Gianfilippo, G.; Donati, C.; Emsley, H.; Forconi, S.; Hopkins, S.; Masotti, L.; et al. Evaluation of C-Reactive Protein Measurement for Assessing the Risk and Prognosis in Ischemic Stroke: A statement for health care professionals from the CRP Pooling Project members. *Stroke* **2005**, *36*, 1316–1329. [CrossRef] [PubMed]
62. Elkind, M.S.V.; Tai, W.; Coates, K.; Paik, M.C.; Sacco, R.L. High-Sensitivity C-Reactive Protein, Lipoprotein-Associated Phospholipase A2, and Outcome After Ischemic Stroke. *Arch. Intern. Med.* **2006**, *166*, 2073–2080. [CrossRef] [PubMed]
63. Muir, K.W.; Weir, C.; Alwan, W.; Squire, I.B.; Lees, K.R. C-Reactive Protein and Outcome After Ischemic Stroke. *Stroke* **1999**, *30*, 981–985. [CrossRef] [PubMed]
64. Gill, R.; Kemp, J.A.; Sabin, C.; Pepys, M.B. Human C-Reactive Protein Increases Cerebral Infarct Size after Middle Cerebral Artery Occlusion in Adult Rats. *J. Cereb. Blood Flow Metab.* **2004**, *24*, 1214–1218. [CrossRef] [PubMed]
65. Liu, F.; Li, L.; Xu, M.; Wu, J.; Luo, D.; Zhu, Y.; Li, B.; Song, X.; Zhou, X. Prognostic value of interleukin-6, C-reactive protein, and procalcitonin in patients with COVID-19. *J. Clin. Virol.* **2020**, *127*, 104370. [CrossRef]
66. Mueller, A.A.; Tamura, T.; Crowley, C.P.; DeGrado, J.R.; Haider, H.; Jezmir, J.L.; Keras, G.; Penn, E.H.; Massaro, A.F.; Kim, E.Y. Inflammatory Biomarker Trends Predict Respiratory Decline in COVID-19 Patients. *Cell Rep. Med.* **2020**, *1*, 100144. [CrossRef]
67. Ruan, Q.; Yang, K.; Wang, W.; Jiang, L.; Song, J. Clinical predictors of mortality due to COVID-19 based on an analysis of data of 150 patients from Wuhan, China. *Intensive Care Med.* **2020**, *46*, 846–848. [CrossRef]
68. Shang, W.; Dong, J.; Ren, Y.; Tian, M.; Li, W.; Hu, J.; Li, Y. The value of clinical parameters in predicting the severity of COVID-19. *J. Med. Virol.* **2020**, *92*, 2188–2192. [CrossRef]
69. Tan, C.; Huang, Y.; Shi, F.; Tan, K.; Ma, Q.; Chen, Y.; Jiang, X.; Li, X. C-reactive protein correlates with computed tomographic findings and predicts severe COVID-19 early. *J. Med. Virol.* **2020**, *92*, 856–862. [CrossRef]
70. Nienhold, R.; Ciani, Y.; Koelzer, V.H.; Tzankov, A.; Haslbauer, J.D.; Menter, T.; Schwab, N.; Henkel, M.; Frank, A.; Zsikla, V.; et al. Two distinct immunopathological profiles in autopsy lungs of COVID-19. *Nat. Commun.* **2020**, *11*, 5086. [CrossRef]
71. Torzewski, M. C-reactive Protein: Friend or Foe? Evidence from Phylogeny. *Front. Cardiovasc. Med.* 2022; in press.
72. Smilowitz, N.R.; Nguy, V.; Aphinyanaphongs, Y.; Newman, J.D.; Xia, Y.; Reynolds, H.R.; Hochman, J.S.; Fishman, G.I.; Berger, J.S. Multiple Biomarker Approach to Risk Stratification in COVID-19. *Circulation* **2021**, *143*, 1338–1340. [CrossRef] [PubMed]
73. Velavan, T.P.; Meyer, C.G. Mild versus severe COVID-19: Laboratory markers. *Int. J. Infect. Dis.* **2020**, *95*, 304–307. [CrossRef] [PubMed]
74. Wu, Z.; McGoogan, J.M. Characteristics of and Important Lessons From the Coronavirus Disease 2019 (COVID-19) Outbreak in China: Summary of a Report of 72,314 Cases From the Chinese Center for Disease Control and Prevention. *JAMA* **2020**, *323*, 1239–1242. [CrossRef]
75. Bhatraju, P.K.; Ghassemieh, B.J.; Nichols, M.; Kim, R.; Jerome, K.R.; Nalla, A.K.; Greninger, A.L.; Pipavath, S.; Wurfel, M.M.; Evans, L.; et al. COVID-19 in Critically Ill Patients in the Seattle Region—Case Series. *N. Engl. J. Med.* **2020**, *382*, 2012–2022. [CrossRef]
76. Mehta, P.; McAuley, D.F.; Brown, M.; Sanchez, E.; Tattersall, R.S.; Manson, J.J.; on behalf of the HLH Across Speciality Collaboration, UK. COVID-19: Consider cytokine storm syndromes and immunosuppression. *Lancet* **2020**, *395*, 1033–1034. [CrossRef]
77. Mosquera-Sulbaran, J.A.; Pedreañez, A.; Carrero, Y.; Callejas, D. C-reactive protein as an effector molecule in COVID-19 pathogenesis. *Rev. Med. Virol.* **2021**, *31*, e2221. [CrossRef]
78. Kayser, S.; Kunze, R.; Sheriff, A. Selective C-reactive protein apheresis for COVID-19 patients suffering from organ damage. *Ther. Apher. Dial.* **2020**, *25*, 251–252. [CrossRef]
79. Pepys, M.B. C-reactive protein predicts outcome in COVID-19: Is it also a therapeutic target? *Eur. Heart J.* **2021**, *42*, 2280–2283. [CrossRef]
80. Ringel, J.; Ramlow, A.; Bock, C.; Sheriff, A. Case Report: C-Reactive Protein Apheresis in a Patient With COVID-19 and Fulminant CRP Increase. *Front. Immunol.* **2021**, *12*, 708101. [CrossRef]
81. Schumann, C.; Heigl, F.; Rohrbach, I.J.; Sheriff, A.; Wagner, L.; Wagner, F.; Torzewski, J. A Report on the First 7 Sequential Patients Treated Within the C-Reactive Protein Apheresis in COVID (CACOV) Registry. *Am. J. Case Rep.* **2021**, *23*, e935263. [CrossRef] [PubMed]
82. Torzewski, J.; Zimmermann, O.; Kayser, S.; Heigl, F.; Wagner, F.; Sheriff, A.; Schumann, C. Successful Treatment of a 39-Year-Old COVID-19 Patient with Respiratory Failure by Selective C-Reactive Protein Apheresis. *Am. J. Case Rep.* **2021**, *22*, e932964. [CrossRef] [PubMed]
83. Szalai, A.J.; McCrory, M.A.; Xing, N.; Hage, F.G.; Miller, A.; Oparil, S.; Chen, Y.-F.; Mazzone, M.; Early, R.; Henry, S.P.; et al. Inhibiting C-Reactive Protein for the Treatment of Cardiovascular Disease: Promising Evidence from Rodent Models. *Mediat. Inflamm.* **2014**, *2014*, 353614. [CrossRef] [PubMed]
84. Pepys, M.B.; Hirschfield, G.; Tennent, G.A.; Gallimore, J.R.; Kahan, M.C.; Bellotti, V.; Hawkins, P.N.; Myers, R.M.; Smith, M.D.; Polara, A.; et al. Targeting C-reactive protein for the treatment of cardiovascular disease. *Nature* **2006**, *440*, 1217–1221. [CrossRef] [PubMed]

85. Kolkhof, P.; Geerts, A.; Schäfer, S.; Torzewski, J. Cardiac glycosides potently inhibit C-reactive protein synthesis in human hepatocytes. *Biochem. Biophys. Res. Commun.* **2010**, *394*, 233–239. [CrossRef] [PubMed]
86. Mattecka, S.; Brunner, P.; Hähnel, B.; Kunze, R.; Vogt, B.; Sheriff, A. PentraSorb C-Reactive Protein: Characterization of the Selective C-Reactive Protein Adsorber Resin. *Ther. Apher. Dial.* **2019**, *23*, 474–481. [CrossRef]
87. Heigl, F.; Pflederer, T.; Klingel, R.; Hettich, R.; Lotz, N.; Reeg, H.; Schettler, V.J.; Roeseler, E.; Grützmacher, P.; Hohenstein, B.; et al. Lipoprotein apheresis in Germany—Still more commonly indicated than implemented. How can patients in need access therapy? *Atheroscler. Suppl.* **2019**, *40*, 23–29. [CrossRef]
88. Grazia, Z.M.; Claudia, S. Effects of selective H.E.L.P. LDL-apheresis on plasma inflammatory markers concentration in severe dyslipidemia: Implication for anti-inflammatory response. *Cytokine* **2011**, *56*, 850–854. [CrossRef]
89. Ries, W.; Sheriff, A.; Heigl, F.; Zimmermann, O.; Garlichs, C.D.; Torzewski, J. "First in Man": Case Report of Selective C-Reactive Protein Apheresis in a Patient with Acute ST Segment Elevation Myocardial Infarction. *Case Rep. Cardiol.* **2018**, *2018*, 4767105. [CrossRef]
90. Ries, W.; Heigl, F.; Garlichs, C.; Sheriff, A.; Torzewski, J. Selective C-Reactive Protein-Apheresis in Patients. *Ther. Apher. Dial.* **2019**, *23*, 570–574. [CrossRef]
91. Sands, B.E.; Katz, S.; Wolf, D.C.; Feagan, B.G.; Wang, T.; Gustofson, L.-M.; Wong, C.; Vandervoort, M.K.; Hanauer, S. A randomised, double-blind, sham-controlled study of granulocyte/monocyte apheresis for moderate to severe Crohn's disease. *Gut* **2012**, *62*, 1288–1294. [CrossRef] [PubMed]
92. Sands, B.E.; Sandborn, W.J.; Feagan, B.; Löfberg, R.; Hibi, T.; Wang, T.; Gustofson, L.; Wong, C.J.; Vandervoort, M.K.; Hanauer, S. A Randomized, Double-Blind, Sham-Controlled Study of Granulocyte/Monocyte Apheresis for Active Ulcerative Colitis. *Gastroenterology* **2008**, *135*, 400–409. [CrossRef] [PubMed]
93. Bosch, T. Recent advances in therapeutic apheresis. *J. Artif. Organs* **2003**, *6*, 1–8. [CrossRef] [PubMed]

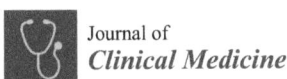

Article

Seven COVID-19 Patients Treated with C-Reactive Protein (CRP) Apheresis

Fabrizio Esposito [1,*], Harald Matthes [2,3,4] and Friedemann Schad [5]

[1] Intensiv-Notfallmedizin und Kardiologie, Gemeinschaftskrankenhaus Havelhöhe, 14089 Berlin, Germany
[2] Gastroenterologie, Gemeinschaftskrankenhaus Havelhöhe, 14089 Berlin, Germany; harald.matthes@charite.de
[3] Medizinischen Klinik für Gastroenterologie, Infektiologie und Rheumatologie, Charité-Universitätsmedizin, 12203 Berlin, Germany
[4] Institut für Sozialmedizin, Epidemiologie und Gesundheitsökonomie, Charité-Universitätsmedizin, 10117 Berlin, Germany
[5] Interdisziplinäre Onkologie und Supportivmedizin, Gemeinschaftskrankenhaus Havelhöhe, 14089 Berlin, Germany; friedemann.schad@havelhoehe.de
* Correspondence: fabrizio.esposito@havelhoehe.de

Abstract: Background: The fulminant course of COVID-19, triggered by severe acute respiratory syndrome coronavirus 2 (SARS-CoV-2), presents with a high mortality rate and still lacks a causative treatment. C-reactive protein (CRP) has been shown to increase dramatically during the disease progression and correlates with deleterious outcomes. Selective CRP apheresis can reduce circulating CRP levels fast and effective. Methods: Seven hospitalized patients with documented severe COVID-19 progression, elevated CRP plasma levels (>100 mg/L) and signs of respiratory failure were treated with CRP apheresis. Two to twelve CRP apheresis sessions were performed generally in 24 h time intervals and depending on CRP plasma levels. Results: All patients had comorbidities. CRP apheresis reduced CRP plasma levels by up to 84% within a few hours, without exhibiting side effects in any patient. Despite signs of severe lung infiltration in all patients, only one patient died. The other patients showed improvements within the chest X-ray after CRP apheresis and were able to recover regardless of intubation and/or ECMO (4 patients). All remaining six patients were discharged from the hospital in good clinical condition. Conclusions: This case series presents a mortality rate of only 14%, which is dramatically lower than expected from the presented CRP levels as well as comorbidities and ventilation requirements. Our clinical observations regarding the here presented seven patients support the hypothesis that CRP is a candidate to be therapeutically targeted in the early stage of severe COVID-19.

Keywords: blood component removal; C-reactive protein; CRP apheresis; COVID-19; multiple organ failure; pulmonary fibrosis; SARS virus

Citation: Esposito, F.; Matthes, H.; Schad, F. Seven COVID-19 Patients Treated with C-Reactive Protein (CRP) Apheresis. J. Clin. Med. 2022, 11, 1956. https://doi.org/10.3390/jcm11071956

Academic Editor: Ahmed Sheriff

Received: 26 February 2022
Accepted: 26 March 2022
Published: 1 April 2022

Publisher's Note: MDPI stays neutral with regard to jurisdictional claims in published maps and institutional affiliations.

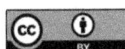

Copyright: © 2022 by the authors. Licensee MDPI, Basel, Switzerland. This article is an open access article distributed under the terms and conditions of the Creative Commons Attribution (CC BY) license (https://creativecommons.org/licenses/by/4.0/).

1. Introduction

C-reactive protein (CRP) is an established biomarker of infection since it was first described in 1930 by Tillet and Francis [1] and can be used as a reliable and fast indicator of the extent of inflammation in the human body. As a classical acute phase protein, CRP rises dramatically within hours of infection or incident and has been shown to activate the complement system via the classical pathway [2] and macrophages via Fcγ-receptors [3,4]. Recently, CRP is not assumed to be only a marker anymore but hypothesized to be an active player in inflammation-induced deleterious tissue processes. This is mainly based on its cytotoxic activity within ischemic and inflamed tissue [5]. After binding to the cell surface, the CRP pentamer may dissociate into monomers suspected to be the pathological agent [6–10]. The question of guilt regarding monomeric or pentameric CRP cannot be clarified by this registry study. Based on the description of the function of the CRP adsorber, we can at least conclude that this medical device adsorbs pentameric CRP [11]. We lack the means to investigate whether it breaks down into the monomer after binding to its target structure.

It has been shown by pathologists [12] that in pulmonary fibrosis, the innate immune system is massively represented, but the adaptive immune system is not. Furthermore, SARS-CoV-2 is hardly detectable. In fact, one would have expected the innate immune system to intervene first and thereafter the adaptive immune system would be activated. With COVID-19, it seems to be the other way around than usual. First, a lot of adaptive immune system can be detected and thereafter the innate immune system causes damage in the lungs.

In the context of the SARS-CoV-2-induced disease COVID-19 it is remarkable that CRP plasma levels rise to an extent similar to bacterial infections [13]. Further, CRP levels correlate with worse prognosis in COVID-19 with an odds ratio of 18.9 [14] and were proven to be a reliable marker for numerous deleterious processes, as, e.g., the need for mechanical ventilation [13,15]. Hence, therapeutically targeting CRP was suggested early on during the pandemic [16,17].

CRP apheresis is an extracorporeal procedure, which decreases CRP plasma levels selectively and with no side effects. Thereby, CRP can finally be targeted therapeutically and specifically [18–21]. It was recently introduced as a potential treatment of severe SARS-CoV-2-induced pneumonia [16,22]. After three case reports describing individual healing attempts [22–24] the "C-reactive protein Apheresis in COVID" (CACOV; DRKS00024376) registry was initiated, which already led to the publication of a case series by another participating center [25]. The seven severe COVID-19 patients treated there survived in good health. Further and based on the results of the CACOV registry, the randomized "C-reactive protein Apheresis for Attenuation of Pulmonary, Myocardial and/or Kidney Injury in COVID-19" (CAPMYKCO; NCT04898062) trial was designed.

From the experience with CRP apheresis in myocardial infarction, we concluded that the earliest possible time for the use of CRP apheresis should be aimed for, which we assume to be in the first 72 h after the onset of severe COVID-19. A publication by Mueller et al. reported that a CRP increase after hospitalization of 13 mg/L within 48 h indicates a poor prognosis including invasive ventilation [13]. The same was shown for CRP levels on admission to the hospital. Here, the threshold value is approximately 146 mg/L. Another publication puts the CRP cutoff value at around 97 mg/L [26]. This report summarizes the treatment of seven COVID-19 patients suffering from severe SARS-CoV-2-induced pneumonia treated by CRP apheresis.

2. Materials and Methods

2.1. CACOV Registry

The CACOV registry is a post market clinical follow up to investigate the reduction of C-reactive protein (CRP) by selective C-reactive protein apheresis in patients with COVID-19 and highly elevated CRP plasma levels. This analysis includes the first seven patients with severe SARS-CoV-2-induced pneumonia and signs of respiratory failure who exceeded CRP plasma levels of 100 mg/L and who could be subjected to CRP apheresis in the early phase (first 72 h) of severe COVID-19. Patients were treated between March and May 2021. All patients provided written informed consent. In this registry, the only inclusion criterion is, that the patient with positive PCR-test for SARS-CoV-2 should have elevated CRP and be treated with CRP apheresis. All patients required intensive care.

2.2. CRP Apheresis

A regenerative single adsorbent system was used for CRP apheresis (PentraSorb® CRP; Pentracor GmbH, Hennigsdorf, Germany). Apheresis is performed in cycles, alternating between loading the adsorber with patient plasma and regeneration, which follows a fixed sequence of wash solutions ($\geq$100 mL NaCl, $\geq$60 mL glycine/HCl, $\geq$80 mL PBS and $\geq$80 mL NaCl). The flow of plasma and wash solutions during apheresis was controlled by an automated plasma flow management software module (ADAsorb, medicap clinic GmbH,

Ulrichstein, Germany). Blood collection was performed via central venous access because of the high clotting tendency of COVID-19 patients. Plasma separation was performed with a centrifuge (SpectraOptia, TerumoBCT, Denver, CO, USA). For plasma separation, blood was anticoagulated with 1:15 citrate buffer (Anticoagulant Citrate Dextrose Solution A = ACD-A). Plasma flow through the adsorber was 25 to 40 mL/min. Blood flow ranged from 47 to 90 mL/min. Up to 8000 mL of plasma was processed during the treatments, preferably in cycles (change of loading and regeneration of the adsorber) of 1000 and 500 mL, respectively. For routine monitoring of apheresis, blood was drawn from the extracorporeal circulation before and after each treatment to determine the CRP concentration.

2.3. Ventilation Scheme

In hypoxic patients or SpO2 < 90%, we started oxygen therapy by goggle or mask, high-flow oxygen therapy and later noninvasive ventilation if necessary, taking into account that delay of intubation in the absence of response to non-invasive ventilation (NIV) worsens the prognosis. In parallel, we performed restrictive fluid therapy in circulatory stable patients.

In invasively ventilated patients, we aimed for a protective ventilation strategy with $Vt \leq 6$ mL/kg, driving pressure < 15 cm H_2O, end-inspiratory airway pressure (pInsp) < 28 cm H_2O and the PEEP setting was based on the so-called high-PEEP table. We performed early abdominal positioning with at least 16 h abdominal positioning intervals. In case of refractory hypoxemia, inhalative application of nitric oxide (NO) was performed and recruitment maneuvers were considered, if necessary, after sonography/CT/EIT. In case of persistent hypoxia, after exhaustion of further therapeutic measures, exclusion of contraindications and consultation with relatives regarding the patient's wishes, the use of venovenous extracorporeal membrane oxygenation (ECMO) was performed.

2.4. Contraindications

Liver failure, hepatic insufficiency, as citrate is used as an anticoagulant in the centrifuge for plasma separation. If citrate is not metabolized quickly by the liver, the blood becomes acidic. Therefore, the liver function should be sound.

3. Results

3.1. Patient Characteristics

We used defined criteria for the selection of patients for this case series. Patients had to be diagnosed with the severe course of COVID-19 and the first CRP apheresis had to be performed a maximum 72 h after the onset of this severe course. The severe disease course was defined by the requirement for oxygen supply, a CRP plasma concentration > 100 mg/L, a poor overall condition and visible COVID-19 infiltrates in the chest X-ray/CT.

Patient characteristics are summarized in Table 1. Age, sex, preexisting and concurrent diseases, length of hospital stay (7–75 days), ventilation therapy (exact type indicated) as well as treatment and apheresis data are shown. All seven patients required either non-invasive oxygen supply or invasive ventilation therapy and suffered from concomitant diseases. Six of seven patients suffered from bacterial superinfection during the hospital stay and therefore received antibiotic therapy.

Patients received 2–12 apheresis sessions depending on their CRP concentration and overall condition. CRP depletion rates ranged from 18–84% per session, strongly depending on the processed plasma volume, stage of CRP synthesis (acute phase) and initial concentration (see Figure 1 for detailed kinetics).

Table 1. Patient characteristics. The table shows age, sex, concomitant diseases, respiratory supply, in-hospital length of stay and treatment parameters of all 7 patients. All patients had documented SARS-CoV-2-induced pneumonia and showed signs of respiratory failure. Patient 6 had acute renal failure (AKI) shortly before his demise. F female, M male, HF High Flow, NIV non-invasive ventilation, M ventilation mechanical ventilation, y yes, n no, ECMO extracorporeal membrane oxygenation, Dex Dexamethasone, Col Colchicine, ABs antibiotics, HVL Gemeinschaftskrankenhaus Havelhöhe (our hospital).

Patient Number	Age	Sex	Hospitalized (Days)	Type of Ventilation (Days)	Treatment	CRP Apheresis (n)	CRP Depletion	Processed Plasma Volume	X-ray Improvement after Apheresis	Survival	Preexisting Diseases Adipositas	Diabetes (Type)	Cardiovascular	Other	Concurrent Diseases
1	33	F	7	Nasal cannula (3)	Dex, Col, ABs	2	58–67%	7.5 L	y	y	y	n	y	Factor V Leiden, Factor II Mutation, microcytic anemia	Bacterial s.infection
2	54	F	44	HF and NIV (24) ECMO (19)	ABs	2	69–70%	7.5–8 L	y (1st)	y	y	Type 2	y		Bacterial s.infection
3	69	M	75	HF (3) M ventilation (72)	ABs	12	13–84%	6.5–10 L	y (6th)	y	y	Type 2	y		Bacterial s.infeccion
4	47	M	39 (34 HVL)	HF (1) M ventilation (24)	ABs	7	20–69%	5–10 L	y (2nd)	y	y	n	y		Bacterial s.infection
5	72	F	9	Nasal cannula (8)	Dex, Col	2	71–72%	4–6 L	y (2nd)	y	y	n	n	Alcohol abusement	
6	77	M	13	HF and NIV (7) M Ventilation (5) ECMO (8)	ABs	7	18–71%	7–9 L	y (5th) Then worse until death	n	n	Type 2	y	multimorbid	Bacterial s.infection, AKI
7	53	F	17	Nasal cannula (7) HF (10) ECMO (10)	Dex, Col, ABs	5	15–71%	6–8.5 L	y (5th)	y	n	n	y		Viral hepatitis, Bacterial s.infection
Mean	57.9		29.1			5.3									

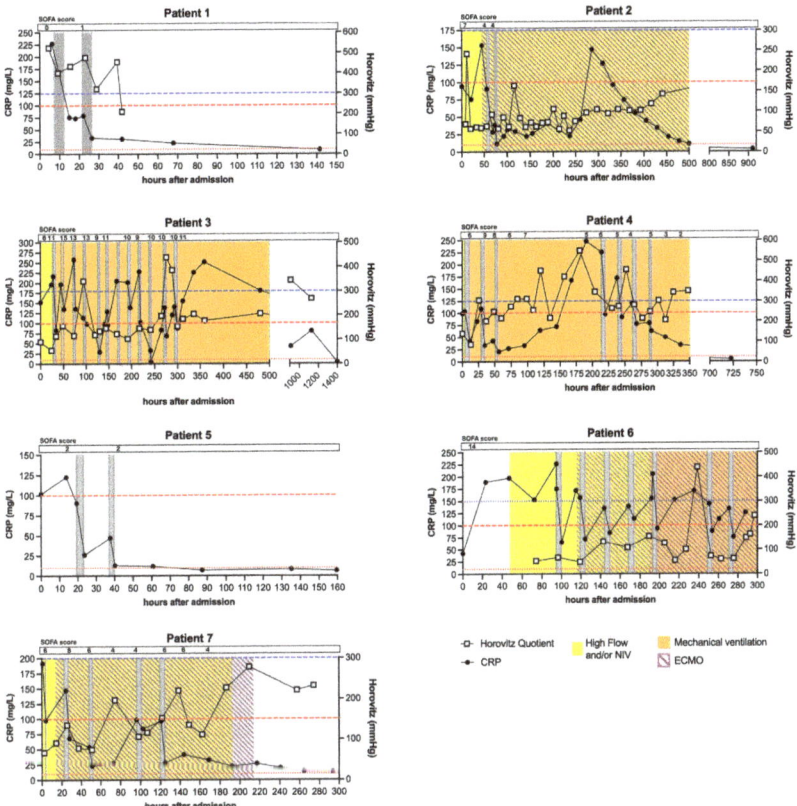

Figure 1. CRP kinetics, Horovitz Quotient and SOFA scores of all patients of the case series. CRP was measured at least every 24 h in all patients during in-hospital stay. Red lines indicate 10 mg/L and 100 mg/L as reference for normal levels and cut-off for severe COVID-19 progression respectively. Blue line indicates 300 mmHg as cut-off for an acute lung injury measured by the Horovitz Quotient. Grey bars indicate apheresis treatments. Ventilation by High Flow or Non-Invasive Ventilation (NIV) is marked in yellow. Mechanical ventilation is marked in orange and extracorporeal membrane oxygenation (ECMO) is marked with purple stripes. No ventilation and nasal cannula are not indicated (for details see Table 1). SOFA scores are displayed at corresponding timepoints. For patient 6 the SOFA score was only determined once.

Only one patient (6) died, all others could be discharged in good clinical condition without the requirement of further ventilation.

3.2. CRP Kinetics

Figure 1 depicts the CRP plasma kinetics of each patient. CRP levels were elevated (>100 mg/L) on admission in all patients except patients 2 and 6, who then showed rising levels within the first 20–50 h after admission. CRP apheresis sessions (grey bars) always led to a pronounced decrease in CRP levels. Patients 1, 4, 5 and 7 were treated with apheresis until CRP declined below 100 mg/L and stayed low. Patients 2 and 3 showed a marked increase in CRP levels after their last apheresis session (~300–350 h after admission), which can be correlated with the diagnosed bacterial superinfection (Procalcitonin levels of other patients in Supplementary Figures S1–S6) and was not treated with CRP apheresis but with antibiotics. CRP levels declined before release. CRP levels re-bound steadily after each CRP apheresis session in patient 6 and could not be maintained below 100 mg/L until the patient unfortunately died.

3.3. X-ray/CT Chest Scans

All patients received an initial chest X-ray/CT upon hospital admission and subsequent follow-up scans during or after their stay as follow up, depending on ventilation interventions and overall condition. The time between scans varied from 5 to 115 days.

All surviving patients showed improvements within the follow-up X-ray scans after apheresis sessions (Figure 2). Even patient 6 initially showed lung infiltration improvement after the 5th apheresis session, before deteriorating to multi-organ failure and death.

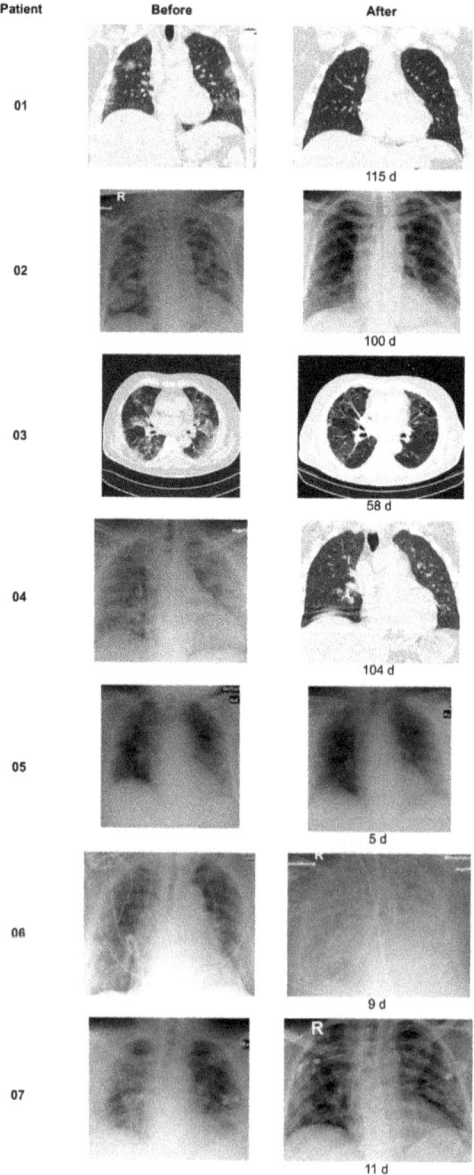

Figure 2. X-ray/CT chest scans. Chest scans were performed before and after treatment/as follow up. The time (days) between the different scans is indicated at the second chest scan.

3.4. Respiratory and Laboratory Parameters

Figure 3 summarizes respiratory parameters in one representative patient (patient 4), Figure 4 summarizes other laboratory results of the same patient.

All patients except patient 6 markedly improved their respiratory parameters during hospitalization (Figure 3). Patient 4 specifically showed metabolic alkalosis (elevated pH and elevated HCO_3^-). He was mechanically ventilated for 24 days (~150–570 h after admission) and showed elevated lactate levels, which normalized over time.

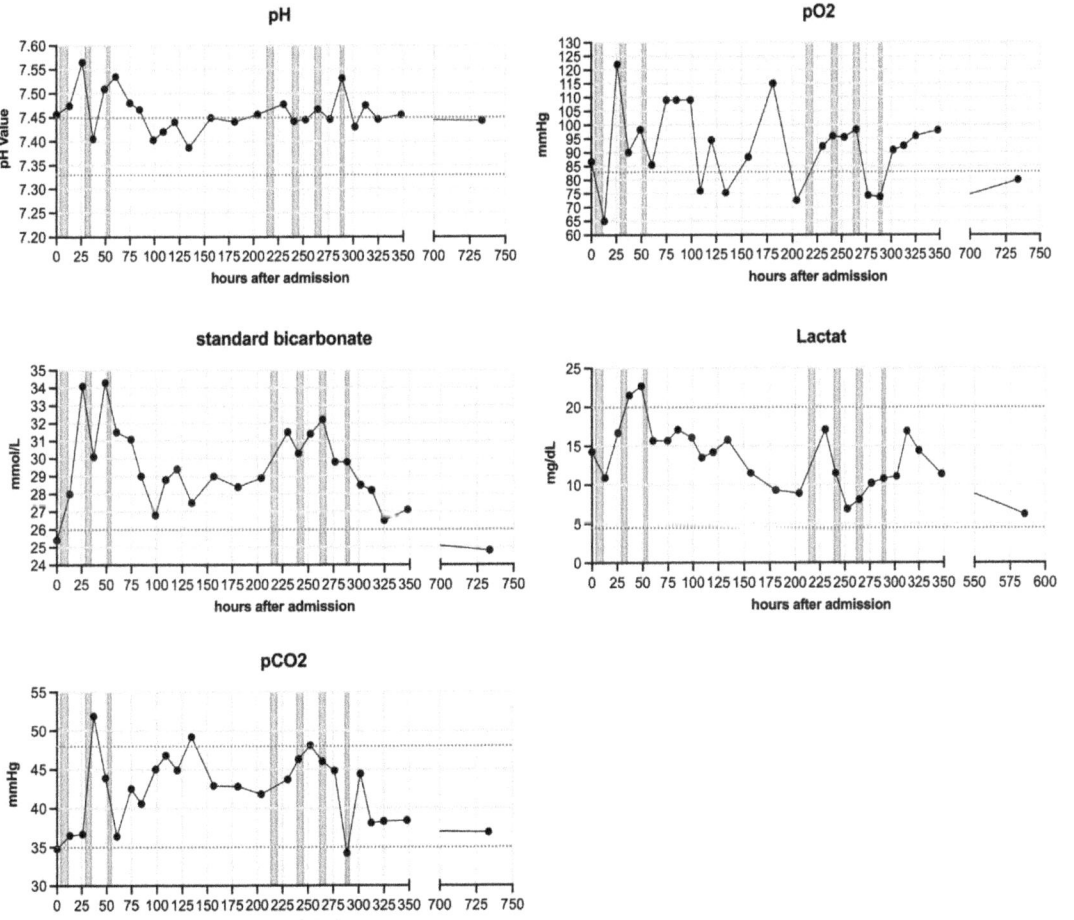

Figure 3. Respiratory parameters of one patient (patient 4). pH, standard HCO_3^-, lactate, arterial pCO_2 and pO_2 were measured regularly for each patient and are depicted here representatively for patient 4. Blue lines indicate minimum baseline and red lines maximum baseline for each normal range. Grey bars indicate apheresis treatments.

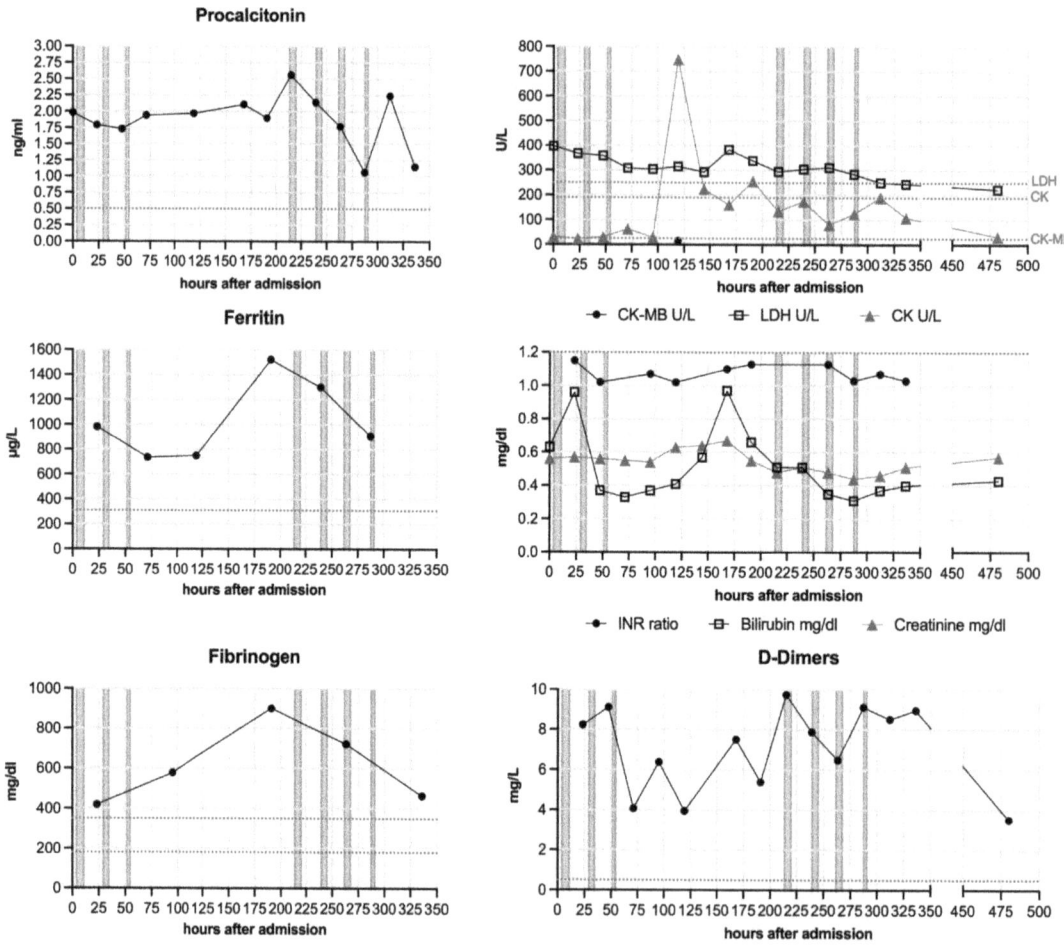

Figure 4. Other laboratory parameters of one patient (patient 4). Procalcitonin, CK-MB, CK, LDH, Ferritin, INR ratio, Bilirubin, Creatinine, Fibrinogen and D-Dimers were measured regularly for each patient and are depicted here representatively for patient 4. Blue lines indicate minimum baseline and red lines maximum baseline for each normal range. Grey bars indicate apheresis treatments.

The other laboratory values (Figure 4) included Procalcitonin, which was elevated in all patients except patient 5, who solely did not receive antibiotic treatment. Four patients had a laboratory constellation of infections at or shortly after admission. Therefore, they were not treated by immunomodulation and immunosuppression. Other parameters (Ferritin, Fibrinogen, D-Dimers, LDH and CK) were also elevated in numerous patients (including 4), but decreased during the hospital stay and were normal upon discharge. Only patient 6 developed signs of multiple organ failure showing rising levels of Bilirubin, Creatinine, LDH and Procalcitonin as well as a severe acidosis. Patient 6 had a SOFA score of 14 at admission to our ICU.

3.5. Control Cohort

At the start of the CACOV registry, we had treated 30 severe COVID-19 patients according to the valid guidelines. Of this cohort, three developed CRP < 100 mg/L. All of them survived. The other 27 developed CRP > 100 mg/L. Thirteen of them died which is 48%.

4. Discussion

The severe course of COVID-19, with its high mortality rate, is fundamentally caused by an excessive immune response, often-called cytokine storm, which mediates the destruction of mainly pulmonary tissue [27,28]. CRP has been established as one of the key effector molecules of this process [5,15,29]. A recent review outlines that and how CRP provides for the disposal of hypoxic cells [5]. This finding is supported by the CRP apheresis after AMI-1 (CAMI-1) clinical trial [18–21]. The CAMI-1 trial clearly and significantly demonstrates, based on results in the control group, that the more CRP the patient synthesizes, the greater the damage to the heart (infarct size, ejection fraction, wall motility). It has been described that this is a dose-dependent effect. Therefore, we suspected that reducing its circulating levels is the next logical step in order to inhibit the deleterious destruction of lung cells, which could recover during ventilation and with more time. CRP apheresis presents the first therapeutic opportunity to target CRP selectively and quickly.

Three COVID-19 patients have been treated with CRP apheresis as individual healing attempts before [22–24]. Subsequently, the CACOV registry started and is running at several centers throughout Germany. Here, we publish a case series of seven patients, with the following characteristics.

All patients reported here were diagnosed with the severe course of COVID-19 and CRP apheresis was initiated within 72 h of this onset. Further, CRP serum levels exceeded 100 mg/L. CRP apheresis significantly decreased the elevated CRP plasma levels in all seven patients, which supports the efficacy of this therapy and is in line with all patients treated with CRP apheresis so far [19–24]. All patients exhibited signs of respiratory or metabolic alkalosis, which is known to occur in COVID-19 [30].

Apart from one patient (6), who unfortunately died of organ failure 14 days after hospital admission, all patients recovered from COVID-19 and could be discharged in good clinical condition after 2–12 CRP apheresis sessions.

All patients besides patient 5 showed elevated Procalcitonin levels and had to be treated with antibiotics. Further, three patients received Dexamethasone/Colchicine upon hospital admission (Table 1), which is known to lower CRP plasma levels to a certain extent for a short period. However, this was not robustly visible within the individual CRP kinetics (Figure 1) and the performed CRP apheresis, with an up to 84% reduction within hours, was definitely more efficient in decreasing CRP plasma levels.

Based on the existing literature and our results, we assume that fluid retention in the lungs and the hypoxia induced by it provide for the induction of CRP [5,23]. The CRP kinetics then depends on the kinetics of the fluid retention and also on the kinetics of the disappearance of the fluid.

Focusing on the CRP kinetics, all patients depicted maximum CRP levels over 120 mg/L. The significant correlation of the increase in CRP as well as the maximum CRP amount with mortality has been widely established so far [14,31–33]. In detail, in one study a 108 mg/L CRP cut-off led to a higher mortality of 32% vs. 18% [15]. In another report, a maximum CRP serum concentration of >100 mg/L was associated with either progressive or severe COVID-19 with a mortality of up to 59% vs. 4% in the mild group (<100 mg/L) [13]. In our in-house control cohort, 48% of severe COVID-19 patients which developed CRP > 100 mg/L died. However, in our case series, the mortality rate was only 14% and thereby dramatically lower than expected from the presented CRP levels as well as co-morbidities and ventilation requirements. All of them are in good health in February 2022 and, therefore, at least 9 months after discharge from the hospital. This is remarkable, as reports from Germany [34] and the US [35] showed that there is a significantly increased risk for mortality over the next 6 or 12 months, respectively. Our clinical observations regarding the here presented seven patients support the hypothesis that CRP should be therapeutically targeted in COVID-19.

4.1. Limitations

In order to conclusively prove that CRP apheresis is the therapy of choice in severe COVID-19 courses, randomized controlled trials are urgently needed.

4.2. Conclusions

Our data support the hypothesis that the damage to the lung caused in severe COVID-19 appears to result primarily from excessive CRP-mediated disposal of oxygen-depleted lung areas. CRP apheresis starting early after patient admission, may potentially be an effective treatment COVID-19 and save lung tissue. Additional registry data and randomized controlled clinical trials are required.

Supplementary Materials: The following supporting information can be downloaded at: https://www.mdpi.com/article/10.3390/jcm11071956/s1, Figures S1–S6: Respiratory and laboratory parameters of Patient 1–3 and 5–7.

Author Contributions: F.E. acquired and analyzed the data and wrote the manuscript. H.M. and F.S. edited the manuscript. All authors have read and agreed to the published version of the manuscript.

Funding: The CACOV-registry is supported by Pentracor GmbH, Hennigsdorf, Germany. Pentracor is the manufacturer of the PentraSorb. The effort required to complete a CRF for CACOV patients is compensated.

Institutional Review Board Statement: The studies involving human participants were reviewed and approved by Ethik-Kommission der Ärztekammer Berlin No. 28/21. All patients gave their written informed consent.

Informed Consent Statement: Informed consent was obtained from all subjects involved in the study.

Data Availability Statement: The original contributions presented in the study are included in the article/Supplementary Materials, further inquiries can be directed to the corresponding author.

Acknowledgments: We gratefully acknowledge Anja Ramlow and Charlene Edge, Pentracor GmbH, Germany, for organizing and performing CRP apheresis.

Conflicts of Interest: These patients were treated within the CACOV registry. The manufacturer Pentracor GmbH is supposed to pay a fee as agreed with the ethics committee for the effort to complete the CRFs. The authors declare that the research was conducted in the absence of any other commercial or financial relationships that could be construed as a potential conflict of interest.

References

1. Tillett, W.S.; Francis, T. Serological Reactions in Pneumonia with a Non-Protein Somatic Fraction of Pneumococcus. *J. Exp. Med.* **1930**, *52*, 561–571. [CrossRef] [PubMed]
2. Kaplan, M.H.; Volanakis, J.E. Interaction of C-reactive protein complexes with the complement system. I. Consumption of human complement associated with the reaction of C-reactive protein with pneumococcal C-polysaccharide and with the choline phosphatides, lecithin and sphingomyelin. *J. Immunol.* **1974**, *112*, 2135–2147. [PubMed]
3. Bharadwaj, D.; Stein, M.P.; Volzer, M.; Mold, C.; Du Clos, T.W. The major receptor for C-reactive protein on leukocytes is fcgamma receptor II. *J. Exp. Med.* **1999**, *190*, 585–590. [CrossRef] [PubMed]
4. Manolov, D.E.; Rocker, C.; Hombach, V.; Nienhaus, G.U.; Torzewski, J. Ultrasensitive confocal fluorescence microscopy of C-reactive protein interacting with FcgammaRIIa. *Arterioscler. Thromb. Vasc. Biol.* **2004**, *24*, 2372–2377. [CrossRef] [PubMed]
5. Sheriff, A.; Kayser, S.; Brunner, P.; Vogt, B. C-Reactive Protein Triggers Cell Death in Ischemic Cells. *Front. Immunol.* **2021**, *12*, 630430. [CrossRef]
6. Boncler, M.; Wu, Y.; Watala, C. The Multiple Faces of C-Reactive Protein-Physiological and Pathophysiological Implications in Cardiovascular Disease. *Molecules* **2019**, *24*, 2062. [CrossRef]
7. Braig, D.; Nero, T.L.; Koch, H.-G.; Kaiser, B.; Wang, X.; Thiele, J.R.; Morton, C.J.; Zeller, J.; Kiefer, J.; Potempa, L.A.; et al. Transitional changes in the CRP structure lead to the exposure of proinflammatory binding sites. *Nat. Commun.* **2017**, *8*, 14188. [CrossRef]
8. McFadyen, J.D.; Kiefer, J.; Braig, D.; Loseff-Silver, J.; Potempa, L.A.; Eisenhardt, S.U.; Peter, K. Dissociation of C-Reactive Protein Localizes and Amplifies Inflammation: Evidence for a Direct Biological Role of C-Reactive Protein and Its Conformational Changes. *Front. Immunol.* **2018**, *9*, 1351. [CrossRef]
9. Thiele, J.R.; Zeller, J.; Bannasch, H.; Stark, G.B.; Peter, K.; Eisenhardt, S.U. Targeting C-Reactive Protein in Inflammatory Disease by Preventing Conformational Changes. *Mediat. Inflamm.* **2015**, *2015*, 372432. [CrossRef]

10. Sproston, N.R.; Ashworth, J.J. Role of C-Reactive Protein at Sites of Inflammation and Infection. *Front. Immunol.* **2018**, *9*, 754. [CrossRef]
11. Mattecka, S.; Brunner, P.; Hähnel, B.; Kunze, R.; Vogt, B.; Sheriff, A. PentraSorb C-Reactive Protein: Characterization of the Selective C-Reactive Protein Adsorber Resin. *Ther. Apher. Dial.* **2019**, *23*, 474–481. [CrossRef] [PubMed]
12. Nienhold, R.; Ciani, Y.; Koelzer, V.H.; Tzankov, A.; Haslbauer, J.D.; Menter, T.; Schwab, N.; Henkel, M.; Frank, A.; Zsikla, V.; et al. Two distinct immunopathological profiles in autopsy lungs of COVID-19. *Nat. Commun.* **2020**, *11*, 5086. [CrossRef] [PubMed]
13. Mueller, A.A.; Tamura, T.; Crowley, C.P.; DeGrado, J.R.; Haider, H.; Jezmir, J.L.; Keras, G.; Penn, E.H.; Massaro, A.F.; Kim, E.Y. Inflammatory Biomarker Trends Predict Respiratory Decline in COVID-19 Patients. *Cell Rep. Med.* **2020**, *1*, 100144. [CrossRef]
14. Parimoo, A.; Biswas, A.; Baitha, U.; Gupta, G.; Pandey, S.; Ranjan, P.; Gupta, V.; Barman Roy, D.; Prakash, B.; Wig, N. Dynamics of Inflammatory Markers in Predicting Mortality in COVID-19. *Cureus* **2021**, *13*, e19080. [CrossRef]
15. Smilowitz, N.R.; Kunichoff, D.; Garshick, M.; Shah, B.; Pillinger, M.; Hochman, J.S.; Berger, J.S. C-reactive protein and clinical outcomes in patients with COVID-19. *Eur. Heart J.* **2021**, *42*, 2270–2279. [CrossRef]
16. Kayser, S.; Kunze, R.; Sheriff, A. Selective C-reactive protein apheresis for Covid-19 patients suffering from organ damage. *Ther. Apher. Dial.* **2021**, *25*, 251–252. [CrossRef] [PubMed]
17. Pepys, M.B. C-reactive protein predicts outcome in COVID-19: Is it also a therapeutic target? *Eur. Heart J.* **2021**, *42*, 2280–2283. [CrossRef]
18. Sheriff, A.; Schindler, R.; Vogt, B.; Abdel-Aty, H.; Unger, J.K.; Bock, C.; Gebauer, F.; Slagman, A.; Jerichow, T.; Mans, D.; et al. Selective apheresis of C-reactive protein: A new therapeutic option in myocardial infarction? *J. Clin. Apher.* **2015**, *30*, 15–21. [CrossRef]
19. Ries, W.; Sheriff, A.; Heigl, F.; Zimmermann, O.; Garlichs, C.D.; Torzewski, J. "First in Man": Case Report of Selective C-Reactive Protein Apheresis in a Patient with Acute ST Segment Elevation Myocardial Infarction. *Case Rep. Cardiol.* **2018**, *2018*, 4767105. [CrossRef]
20. Ries, W.; Heigl, F.; Garlichs, C.; Sheriff, A.; Torzewski, J. Selective C-Reactive Protein-Apheresis in Patients. *Ther. Apher. Dial.* **2019**, *23*, 570–574. [CrossRef]
21. Ries, W.; Torzewski, J.; Heigl, F.; Pfluecke, C.; Kelle, S.; Darius, H.; Ince, H.; Mitzner, S.; Nordbeck, P.; Butter, C.; et al. C-Reactive Protein Apheresis as Anti-inflammatory Therapy in Acute Myocardial Infarction: Results of the CAMI-1 Study. *Front. Cardiovasc. Med.* **2021**, *8*, 155. [CrossRef] [PubMed]
22. Torzweski, J.; Heigl, F.; Zimmermann, O.; Wagner, F.; Schumann, C.; Hettich, R.; Bock, C.; Kayser, S.; Sheriff, A. First-in-man: Case report of Selective C-reactive Protein Apheresis in a Patient with SARS-CoV-2 Infection. *Am. J. Case Rep.* **2020**, *21*, e925020. [CrossRef] [PubMed]
23. Ringel, J.; Ramlow, A.; Bock, C.; Sheriff, A. Case Report: C-Reactive Protein Apheresis in a Patient with COVID-19 and Fulminant CRP Increase. *Front. Immunol.* **2021**, *12*, 3140. [CrossRef] [PubMed]
24. Torzewski, J.; Zimmermann, O.; Kayser, S.; Heigl, F.; Wagner, F.; Sheriff, A.; Schumann, C. Successful Treatment of a 39-Year-Old COVID-19 Patient with Respiratory Failure by Selective C-Reactive Protein Apheresis. *Am. J. Case Rep.* **2021**, *22*, e932964. [CrossRef] [PubMed]
25. Schumann, C.; Heigl, F.; Rohrbach, I.J.; Sheriff, A.; Wagner, L.; Wagner, F.; Torzewski, J. A Report on the First 7 Sequential Patients Treated Within the C-Reactive Protein Apheresis in COVID (CACOV) Registry. *Am. J. Case Rep.* **2022**, *23*, e935263. [CrossRef]
26. Herold, T.; Jurinovic, V.; Arnreich, C.; Lipworth, B.J.; Hellmuth, J.C.; von Bergwelt-Baildon, M.; Klein, M.; Weinberger, T. Elevated levels of IL-6 and CRP predict the need for mechanical ventilation in COVID-19. *J. Allergy Clin. Immunol.* **2020**, *146*, 128–136.e124. [CrossRef]
27. Cappanera, S.; Palumbo, M.; Kwan, S.H.; Priante, G.; Martella, L.A.; Saraca, L.M.; Sicari, F.; Vernelli, C.; Di Giuli, C.; Andreani, P.; et al. When Does the Cytokine Storm Begin in COVID-19 Patients? A Quick Score to Recognize It. *J. Clin. Med.* **2021**, *10*, 297. [CrossRef]
28. Nadeem, R.; Elhoufi, A.M.; Iqbal, N.E.; Obaida, Z.A.; Elgohary, D.M.; Singh, M.K.; Zoraey, S.F.; Abdalla, R.M.; Eltayeb, S.Y.; Danthi, C.S.; et al. Prediction of Cytokine Storm and Mortality in Patients with COVID-19 Admitted to ICU: Do Markers Tell the Story? *Dubai Med. J.* **2021**, *4*, 142–150. [CrossRef]
29. Mosquera-Sulbaran, J.A.; Pedreañez, A.; Carrero, Y.; Callejas, D. C-reactive protein as an effector molecule in Covid-19 pathogenesis. *Rev. Med. Virol.* **2021**, *31*, e2221. [CrossRef]
30. Wu, C.; Wang, G.; Zhang, Q.; Yu, B.; Lv, J.; Zhang, S.; Wu, G.; Wu, S.; Zhong, Y. Association Between Respiratory Alkalosis and the Prognosis of COVID-19 Patients. *Front. Med.* **2021**, *8*, 564635. [CrossRef]
31. Ali, N. Elevated level of C-reactive protein may be an early marker to predict risk for severity of COVID-19. *J. Med. Virol.* **2020**, *92*, 2409–2411. [CrossRef] [PubMed]
32. Sharifpour, M.; Rangaraju, S.; Liu, M.; Alabyad, D.; Nahab, F.B.; Creel-Bulos, C.M.; Jabaley, C.S.; Emory, C.-Q.; Clinical Research, C. C-Reactive protein as a prognostic indicator in hospitalized patients with COVID-19. *PLoS ONE* **2020**, *15*, e0242400. [CrossRef] [PubMed]
33. Villoteau, A.; Asfar, M.; Otekpo, M.; Loison, J.; Gautier, J.; Annweiler, C.; GERIA-COVID Study Group. Elevated C-reactive protein in early COVID-19 predicts worse survival among hospitalized geriatric patients. *PLoS ONE* **2021**, *16*, e0256931. [CrossRef] [PubMed]

34. Günster, C.; Busse, R.; Spoden, M.; Rombey, T.; Schillinger, G.; Hoffmann, W.; Weber-Carstens, S.; Schuppert, A.; Karagiannidis, C. 6-month mortality and readmissions of hospitalized COVID-19 patients: A nationwide cohort study of 8679 patients in Germany. *PLoS ONE* **2021**, *16*, e0255427. [CrossRef]
35. Mainous, A.G., III; Rooks, B.J.; Wu, V.; Orlando, F.A. COVID-19 Post-acute Sequelae Among Adults: 12 Month Mortality Risk. *Front. Med.* **2021**, *8*, 778434. [CrossRef]

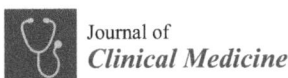

Article

Cardiac Glycosides Lower C-Reactive Protein Plasma Levels in Patients with Decompensated Heart Failure: Results from the Single-Center C-Reactive Protein-Digoxin Observational Study (C-DOS)

Myron Zaczkiewicz [1,*], Katharina Kostenzer [1], Matthias Graf [1], Benjamin Mayer [2], Oliver Zimmermann [1] and Jan Torzewski [1]

1. Cardiovascular Center Oberallgäu-Kempten, 87439 Kempten, Germany; katha_789@yahoo.de (K.K.); matthias.graf@klinikverbund-allgaeu.de (M.G.); oliver.zimmermann@klinikverbund-allgaeu.de (O.Z.); jan.torzewski@klinikverbund-allgaeu.de (J.T.)
2. Institute of Epidemiology and Medical Biometry, University of Ulm, 89081 Ulm, Germany; benjamin.mayer@uni-ulm.de
* Correspondence: myron.zaczkiewicz@klinikverbund-allgaeu.de; Tel.: +49-8323-910-8950

Abstract: Recent randomized controlled multi-center trials JUPITER, CANTOS and COLCOT impressively demonstrated the effect of anti-inflammatory therapy on secondary prevention of cardiovascular events. These studies also rapidly re-vitalized the question of whether the C-reactive protein (CRP), the prototype human acute phase protein, is actively involved in atherosclerosis and its sequelae. Direct CRP inhibition may indeed improve the specificity and effectiveness of anti-inflammatory intervention. In the present paper, we report on the final results of our single-center C-reactive protein-Digoxin Observational Study (C-DOS). Methods and Results: Based on the experimental finding that cardiac glycosides potently inhibit hepatic CRP synthesis on the transcriptional level in vitro, 60 patients with decompensated heart failure, NYHA III–IV, severely reduced Left Ventricular Ejection Fraction (LVEF < 40%), and elevated CRP plasma levels were treated by either digoxin + conventional heart failure therapy (30 patients) or by conventional heart failure therapy alone (30 patients). Plasma CRP levels in both groups were assessed for 21 d. Plasma CRP levels on d1, d3 and d21 were compared by regression analysis. CRP levels d21–d1 significantly declined in both groups. Notably, comparative CRP reduction d21–d3 in digoxin versus the control group also revealed borderline significance ($p = 0.051$). Conclusions: This small observational trial provides the first piece of evidence that cardiac glycosides may inhibit CRP synthesis in humans. In case of further pharmacological developments, cardiac glycosides may emerge as lead compounds for chemical modification in order to improve the potency, selectivity and pharmacokinetics of CRP synthesis inhibition in cardiovascular disease.

Keywords: CRP; CRP synthesis inhibition; cardiovascular disease

Citation: Zaczkiewicz, M.; Kostenzer, K.; Graf, M.; Mayer, B.; Zimmermann, O.; Torzewski, J. Cardiac Glycosides Lower C-Reactive Protein Plasma Levels in Patients with Decompensated Heart Failure: Results from the Single-Center C-Reactive Protein-Digoxin Observational Study (C-DOS). *J. Clin. Med.* **2022**, *11*, 1762. https://doi.org/10.3390/jcm11071762

Academic Editors: Ahmed Sheriff and Massimo Iacoviello

Received: 14 February 2022
Accepted: 18 March 2022
Published: 22 March 2022

Publisher's Note: MDPI stays neutral with regard to jurisdictional claims in published maps and institutional affiliations.

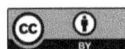

Copyright: © 2022 by the authors. Licensee MDPI, Basel, Switzerland. This article is an open access article distributed under the terms and conditions of the Creative Commons Attribution (CC BY) license (https://creativecommons.org/licenses/by/4.0/).

1. Introduction

The elevated plasma levels of C-reactive protein (CRP), the typical human acute-phase protein, predict future cardiovascular events [1]. Whether this is just an epiphenomenon or whether CRP actively contributes to atherogenesis and its sequelae is still controversial [2,3]. Initial experimental studies were suggestive of this [4–6]. Genetic analyses from Mendelian randomization trials, however, did not support the concept of CRP being actively involved in human cardiovascular disease [7]. Nonetheless, pitfalls in Mendelian randomization have to be taken into account [8]. Furthermore, species differences in CRP biology limit the value of animal models in this particular area of research [2]. Finally, the experimental data from various laboratories were not accurately evaluated [9] and, unfortunately, have shed negative light on the subject in general. There is, however, international consensus that CRP activates the complement system [10] and binds to Fcγ receptors [11] in atherosclerosis [5,6], and thereby may sustain a chronic inflammatory process in the arterial wall.

Recently, the randomized controlled multi-center trials JUPITER [12], CANTOS [13] and COLCOT [14] impressively demonstrated the effect of anti-inflammatory therapy on secondary prevention of cardiovascular events. These studies also rapidly re-vitalized the question of whether CRP is actively involved in atherosclerosis and its sequelae [3,5], because the effect of anti-inflammatory therapy significantly correlates with CRP reduction in each of these trials. Direct CRP inhibition may indeed improve the specificity and effectiveness of anti-inflammatory intervention.

By using a high throughput screening assay in order to analyze the effect of specific classes of pharmacological agents on CRP transcriptions, in 2010 we showed that endogenous and plant-derived inhibitors of the $Na^{(+)}/K^{(+)}$-ATPase, i.e., the cardiac glycosides ouabain, digoxin and digitoxin, inhibit IL-1ß- and IL-6-induced acute phase protein expression in human hepatoma cells and primary human hepatocytes at nanomolar concentrations [15]. Whether this in vitro finding holds true in vivo in humans and is also detected at the CRP plasma level is now being tested in our single-center C-reactive protein-Digoxin Observational Study (C-DOS) [16,17]. A recently published study showed a significant digitoxin-mediated reduction in CRP levels in mice suffering from sepsis, providing a small piece of evidence that cardiac glycosides are also capable of inhibiting CRP synthesis in mice [18].

The primary aim of this study is to evaluate whether CRP plasma levels can be significantly reduced by digoxin, in addition to optimal medical treatment (OMT) in patients with heart failure and reduced Left Ventricular Ejection Fraction (LVEF) admitted to the hospital with acute cardiac decompensation (NYHA class III and IV).

2. Methods

2.1. Study Design

Extensive discussions with the Ethical Review Committee of Ulm University, Ulm, Germany, preceded the C-DOS [16,17]. It was initially designed as a blinded, randomized clinical trial comparing two groups (OMT plus digoxin vs. OMT only). The Ethical Review Committee then advised us to change the design, in order to avoid that final medication (digoxin or not) depends on randomization. Cardiac glycoside treatment was recommended to follow clinical needs only, rather than randomization in a study arm. Obeying the Ethical Review Committee's advice, we designed a prospective observational cohort study, and this design, finally, was approved by the Ethical Review Committee. The patients were recruited in the time span ranging from the end of 2012 until the end of 2019, with an interruption from mid-2016 until mid-2018. This interruption was caused by the surprising pre-emptive review of the study by the Federal Institute for Drugs and Medical Devices of the Federal Republic of Germany (Bundesamt für Arzneimittelsicherheit und Medizinprodukte, BfArM, Bonn, Germany), which examined whether this study was subject to authorization according to the German law ensuring drug safety (Arzneimittelgesetz, AMG; § 4 Abs 23 Satz 1). The review again confirmed that the study was not subject to authorization by the agency, since it was classified by the agency as an observational study on 11 July 2018. This assessment was finally shared by the government of upper Bavaria (Regierung von Oberbayern). Nonetheless, the reglementary process caused an unfortunate interruption in patient recruitment.

2.2. Controls/Comparators

The CRP plasma levels of 30 patients with decompensated heart failure, NYHA III and IV, LVEF < 40%, and OMT plus digoxin were compared to the CRP plasma levels of 30 patients with decompensated heart failure, NYHA III and IV, LVEF < 40%, and OMT alone.

2.3. Inclusion and Exclusion Criteria, Patient Characteristics

Inclusion criteria: age > 18 years; NYHA III and NYHA IV; acute cardiac failure (acute worsening of dyspnoe, and radiological signs of cardiac congestion); and LVEF < 40% in echocardiography (2 observers, Teichholz/Simpson method). The characteristics of the included patients are summarized in Table 1. Exclusion criteria: significant concomitant disease (acute coronary syndrome, infection, antibiotic therapy, acute renal failure, cancer, and autoimmune disease); CRP > 5 mg/dL, leukocyte count > 12,000/µL, body temperature > 38 °C; and AV-block IIII (for digoxin patients).

Table 1. Baseline data and OMT prescribed d1/d21.

Demographic Data	Digoxin Group	Control Group	p-Value
Age (±SD)	71.8 years (±10.6)	73.7 years (±8.6)	n.s.
Sex: male/female	26/4	22/8	n.s.
Clinical data			
NYHA III/IV	26/4	24/6	n.s.
LVEF (±SD)	26.1% (±0.08)	24.5% (±0.06)	n.s.
Ischemic cardiomyopathy (total)	12	11	n.s.
Dilated cardiomyopathy (total)	18	19	n.s.
Clinical chemistry			
Digoxin serum level d1 (±SD)	0.28 µg/L (±0.38)		
Digoxin serum level d21 (±SD)	1.46 µg/L (±0.81)		
Creatinine (±SD)	1.20 mg/dL (±0.35)	1.16 mg/dL (±0.35)	n.s.
Sodium (±SD)	140.53 mmol/L (±3.76)	139.00 mmol/L (±3.38)	n.s.
Potassium (±SD)	4.22 mmol/L (±0.43)	4.34 mmol/L (±0.55)	n.s.
Calcium (±SD)	2.27 mmol/L (±0.12)	2.29 mmol/L (±0.88)	n.s.
proBNP (d1)	8484 pg/mL	8528 pg/mL	n.s.
Red blood cell count (d1)	498 million/µL	464 million/µL	n.s.
ECG rhythm at baseline	Number of patients		
Sinus rhythm	17	26	0.010
Atrial fibrillation	11	4	0.037
Slow VT	1	0	n.s.
Atrial flutter	1	0	n.s.
Class IA medication	Number of patients		
b-blocker (d1/d21)	27/27	26/30	n.s./n.s.
ACE inhibitor (d1/d21)	20/22	24/23	n.s./n.s.
AT1 blocker (d1/d21)	5/5	4/5	n.s./n.s.
Aldosterone antagonist (d1/d21)	19/18	17/28	n.s./0.002

Baseline patient characteristics and heart failure medication on d1 and d21 for the digoxin and control groups (comparison by means of independent t-test and chi-squared test, respectively). n.s. = not significant.

Explanation for the exclusion criteria: an exclusion of CRP > 5 mg/dL, leukocyte count > 12,000/µL, body temperature > 38 °C avoids confounding influence of infection. Due to the expected significant proportion of patients that needed to be excluded, approximately 800 patients were assessed for eligibility. Due to the expected [17] final high drop-out rate of 44%, 107 patients were assigned to the trial. A total of 47 patients were disqualified due to various reasons (see Section 3.1), and only 60 patients were finally included in the trial.

2.4. Outcome Measures

CRP (and digoxin) plasma levels were assessed at d1, d3, d5, d7 and d21 after inclusion. The primary efficacy endpoint was the comparison of CRP plasma level change between the digoxin and control groups during follow-up (d21–d3). D3 was elected under the assumption that an effect of transcriptional CRP synthesis inhibition by cardiac glycosides on CRP plasma levels may be detectable after 3d of digoxin treatment at the earliest. CRP levels were determined via highly sensitive, particle-enhanced immunological turbidity test assays produced by Roche.

The explanation for the follow-up period: CRP plasma half-life in humans is ~19 h. Therapeutic blood concentration of digoxin, with routine saturation, is reached after d3. We assumed that a potential effect of digoxin on CRP synthesis should be visible on d21.

2.5. Methods against Bias

LVEF was echocardiographically analyzed by two investigators via the Teichholz/Simpson method. Multiple regression analysis was used to adjust for potential confounding due to gender, age and cardiac rhythm. CRP plasma levels were assessed by the independent clinical laboratory (Clinic Association Allgäu, Kempten, Germany) via routine CRP measurements. Per protocol analysis of $n = 60$ (30 digoxin vs. 30 control) patients was performed. Blinding was not possible because intervention and control followed clinical needs. Digoxin plasma levels were monitored for safety reasons because of the drug's small therapeutic window.

2.6. Sample Size/Power Calculations

Power calculation was discussed with the Institute of Epidemiology and Medical Biometry of Ulm University. Because no studies exist that investigate the effect of cardiac glycosides on CRP plasma levels, the biometrical classification of the study was "pilot study for subsequent phase III trials". The sample size of 60 patients in total was evaluated as being adequate to apply the aforementioned multiple regression analysis with 3 confounders. The expected drop-out rate was high due to, for example, the acquirement of lung infection following cardiac decompensation, other infectious diseases or bradycardia due to digoxin treatment. There was no database to conduct a formal sample size calculation due to the lack of retrospective trials in the field.

2.7. Feasibility of Treatment

Decompensated heart failure is one of the most common diagnoses on admission in cardiovascular units [19,20]. All admitted patients were screened for inclusion and exclusion criteria. The feasibility and safety of study medication was definitely provided, because cardiac glycosides have been used in cardiac insufficiency for 230 years [21] and, according to the heart failure guidelines, still provide an additive treatment option in NYHA classes III and IV [20,22]. All study participants provided written informed consent.

2.8. Statistical Analysis

After the final data acquisition, all variables were descriptively analyzed. The Wilcoxon singed rank test was used to compare the dx-dy differences per group. The Shapiro–Wilk test was used to check the normal assumption. To assess the efficacy of the investigated treatment scheme, multiple regression analysis was performed. The dependent variable was the difference of CRP plasma level at d21 and d3, the independent variables were the group status (digoxin vs. placebo) and the 3 confounding variables gender, age and cardiac rhythm, i.e., sinus rhythm vs. atrial fibrillation. The level of significance was set to 5% (2-sided). The analysis of all secondary endpoints was conducted in an explorative manner. Analyses concerning safety issues were performed by evaluating the adverse events frequencies in both groups. The expected drop-out rate (50%) was high, due to, for example, the potential acquirement of infection during follow-up. Per protocol analysis of $n = 60$ (30 digoxin vs. 30 control) patients was performed.

3. Results

3.1. Baseline Patient Characteristics, Medication Follow-Up and Drop-Outs

Baseline patient characteristics are summarized in Table 1. The average age was 72.8 years overall with patients in the digoxin group being slightly younger than in the control group (71.8 vs. 73.7 years). A total of 48 men (26 in digoxin group) and 12 women (4 in digoxin group) were enrolled. On admission, 50 patients (26 in digoxin group) were classified as NYHA III and 10 patients (4 in digoxin group) as NYHA IV. LVEF averaged

26.1% in the digoxin group and 24.5% in the control group (25.3% overall). A total of 23 patients suffered from ischemic cardiomyopathy (12 in digoxin vs. 11 in control group), whereas dilated cardiomyopathy (DCM) was diagnosed in 37 patients (18 in digoxin vs. 19 in control group). On admission, ECG showed sinus rhythm in 43 patients (17 in digoxin group) and atrial fibrillation in 15 patients (11 in digoxin group). Atrial flutter and a slow VT were documented in one patient each, both belonging to the digoxin group. Baseline CRP levels on d1 were 1.16 mg/dL in the digoxin group and 0.92 mg/dL in the control group. Further baseline data, including class IA heart failure medication on admission, are shown in Table 1. Class IA heart failure medication is optimized as clinically indicated until d21 in both groups (Table 1) with no statistically significant differences.

Initially, 107 patients were enrolled, of whom 47 patients were not analyzed in this study. This equals a drop-out rate of 43.9%. Patients had to be excluded because of the following reasons: 10 patients (21.7%) withdrew their consent; 9 patients (17.4%) needed antibiotic therapy, which modulates CRP levels itself; 4 (9%) patients needed an ICD implantation, which requests single-shot antibiotic therapy and leads to a rise in CRP levels itself; 3 patients (6.4%) needed other surgical intervention; 2 patients (4.2%) died due to heart failure within the follow-up; and 2 patients (4.3%) were diagnosed with cancer within the follow-up period. Another 2 patients (4.3%) showed complete normalization of LVEF after 21d (main diagnosis: tachycardia-induced cardiomyopathy) and therefore were excluded in line with the study design. The cross over rate was 10.6%, since 5 patients received digoxin due to atrial fibrillation induced tachycardia after they were enrolled in the control group. A total of 5 patients (10.6%) from the digoxin group dropped out due to adverse side effects from digoxin. Another 5 patients (10.6%) were lost in the follow-up; no CRP level could be obtained on d21 after they had been discharged from our hospital.

3.2. CRP Levels in the Digoxin Versus Control Group

In the digoxin group, average CRP levels rose from 1.16 mg/dL on d1 to 1.63 mg/dL on d3 and then dropped steadily to 0.54 mg/dL on d21 (see Figure 1A,B). In the control group, a different course of CRP levels was observed, with the corresponding levels being 0.94 mg/dL on d1, 0.98 mg/dL on d3 and 0.72 mg/dL on d21. Detailed CRP levels are shown in Table 2.

Table 2. CRP levels, normal assumption testing and CRP drop-off comparisons.

	CRP d1 (mg/dL)	CRP d3 (mg/dL)	CRP d5 (mg/dL)	CRP d7 (mg/dL)	CRP d21 (mg/dL)
Digoxin group (±SD)	1.16 (±1.07)	1.62 (±1.80)	1.37 (±1.22)	1.36 (±1.36)	0.54 (±0.67)
Control group (±SD)	0.94 (±0.77)	0.98 (±0.98)	1.23 (±2.19)	1.63 (±2.45)	0.72 (±0.90)
Non-standard distribution	Shapiro–Wilk test	Shapiro–Wilk test			Shapiro–Wilk test
Digoxin group	<0.001	<0.001			<0.001
Control group	<0.001	<0.001			<0.001
	Wilcoxon test	Wilcoxon test	Wilcoxon test		
	Digoxin group	Control group	Group comparison		
d1/d21 (control group)	<0.001	<0.001	0.268		
d3/d21 (control group)	<0.001	0.029	**0.051**		

Average CRP levels and standard deviations on d1, d3, d5, d7 and d21 in both groups, normal assumption testing p-values according to Shapiro–Wilk test for both groups; p-values (Wilcoxon test) for d1/d21 and d3/d21 CRP level comparison within each group; p-values (Wilcoxon test) for group comparison of CRP drop-off from d1/d21 and d3/d21 (**p = 0.051, borderline significance**).

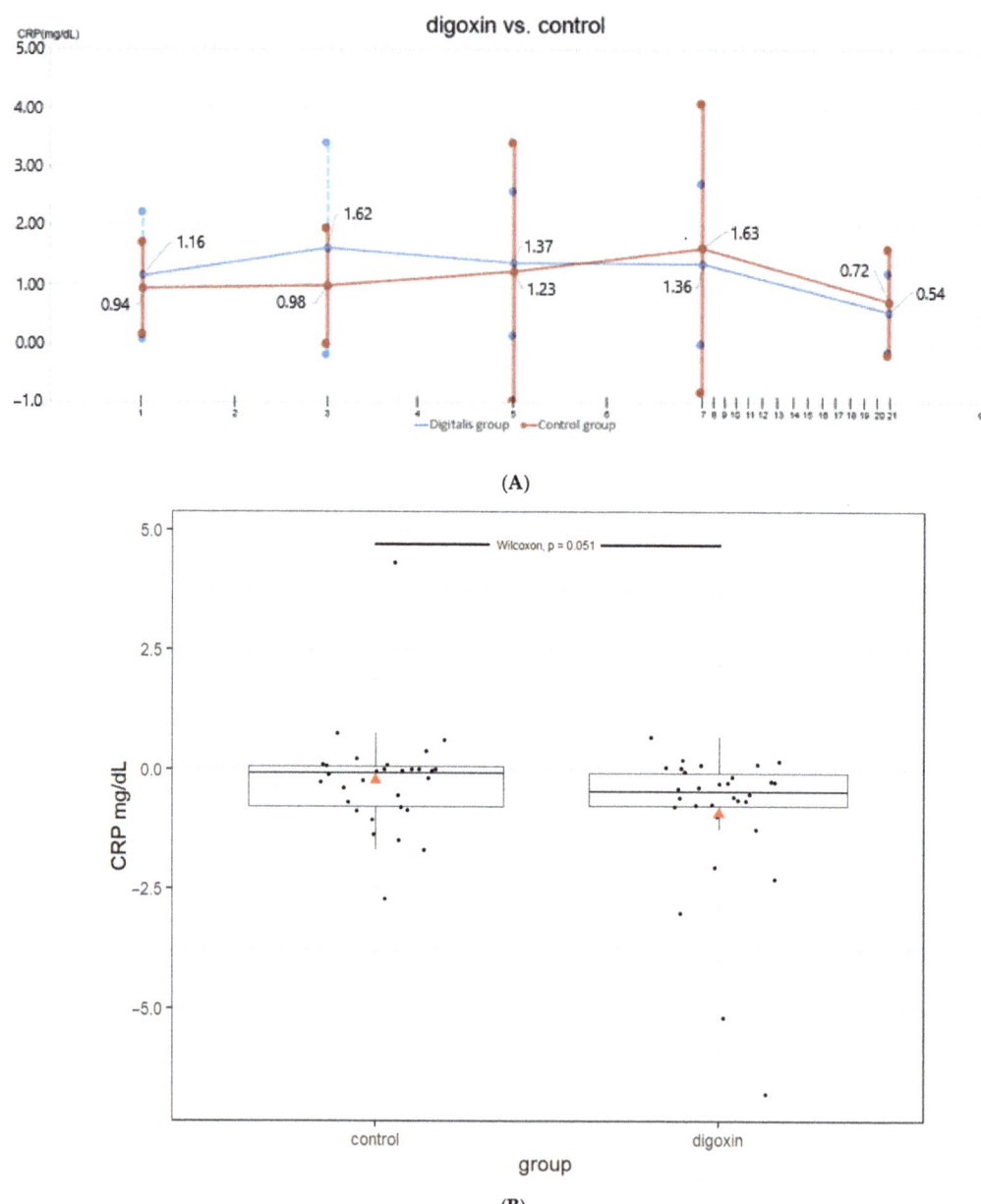

Figure 1. (**A**). Course of mean CRP levels ±SD in the digoxin group and control group (d1 to d21). (**B**) Difference in CRP levels on d21 vs. d3 in the digoxin and control group (box plot: CRP difference d21 vs. d3 digoxin/control group. Triangle = average value, black line = median, upper thin black line = 75. Quantile, lower thin black line = 25. quantile, $p = 0.051$).

As the normal assumption seemed not to be valid, according to the Shapiro–Wilk test, the Wilcoxon signed rank test was performed to compare the within-group differences in the CRP levels. The Wilcoxon ranked sum test was applied in order to compare the difference in the CRP level change (d21–d2) between the digoxin and control group (Table 2). Testing showed a significant decrease in CRP levels within the control as well as within the digoxin group from d1 to d21. The group comparison from d21-d1 between the digoxin and control group revealed no statistically significant differences (Table 2). Notably, a comparison of the CRP plasma level decline d21–d3 between both groups revealed borderline statistical significance ($p = 0.051$; Figure 1; Table 2).

4. Discussion

Cardiac glycosides inhibit hepatocellular CRP synthesis in vitro [15]. The aim of C-DOS was to evaluate the effect of cardiac glycosides on human CRP plasma levels in vivo [17]. Digoxin was chosen as an easy-to-handle and easy-to-monitor standard cardiac glycoside for human application [22]. Since therapeutic digoxin plasma levels are commonly reached after 3d of routine saturation and since transcriptional CRP synthesis inhibition likely does not immediately take place following intake, the crucial time points to compare CRP plasma levels were considered to be d21–d3. Digoxin plasma levels in digoxin-treated patients, during this time span, were within the therapeutic range. Due to the standard treatment of heart failure, CRP levels within each group were significantly lower on d21–d1 and d21–d3. Comparing the degree of CRP plasma level reduction for d21–d3 between both groups revealed borderline significance ($p = 0.051$).

4.1. Limitiations

C-DOS is a single-center explorative pilot study—no more, no less. It is not a randomized trial. It is not multi-centric. The number of study participants (30 vs. 30 patients) was low. Additionally, due to a 2-year legal re-evaluation (see above), it took a relatively long time (2012–2019) to recruit these patients. The primary endpoint, i.e., CRP plasma level reduction d21–d3, is of borderline significance ($p = 0.051$) only. The drop-out rate of 46% is (as originally expected) high. In addition, a bystander effect of the OMT and recompensation measures on CRP levels cannot be completely excluded with this study design and the relatively low number of patients enrolled.

4.2. Possible Implications

C-DOS was designed as a single center explorative pilot study. Randomization was not permitted by the Ethical Review Committee because medical therapy in this high mortality disease was intended to follow medical necessity rather than admission to a study arm. The number of study participants followed statistical advice (see Section 2.6). Notably, although the number of study participants is low, the primary endpoint, i.e., comparative CRP plasma level reduction from d21–d3 between the groups, revealed borderline significance ($p = 0.051$). This indeed suggests that the significance level may be attained in a larger trial. A high drop-out rate was expected from the start of the trial [16,17]. It was caused mostly by circumstances coinciding with the underlying disease, since a lot of the initially enrolled patients needed either antibiotic therapy (due to relevant infectious disease) or surgery (for example ICD implantation) that could not be postponed during the follow-up period. Compliance after discharge played a role, too, since our hospitals, being inserted into the German healthcare system, have no means of follow-up in the ambulatory setting.

Digoxin was only prescribed when indicated and no contraindications existed [23]. This resulted in a higher number of patients with atrial fibrillation and atrial flutter in the digoxin group. Since it has been shown that atrial flutter and atrial fibrillation both coincide with higher CRP levels [24], this may be a reason for higher baseline CRP levels in the digoxin group on d1. Atrial fibrillation/flutter as a confounding factor also proved to be of borderline significance (p-value 0.052) in our statistical analysis.

Statins and ACE inhibitors also lower CRP plasma levels, as has been shown in the JUPITER trial [12] and others [25]. In our observational study, however, there was no statistically significant difference between both groups in terms of ACE-inhibitor and statin therapy. Thus, in our study population, an effect of these two drugs on CRP levels may have been ruled out.

4.3. Context of C-DOS

CANTOS [13] showed a 15% relative risk reduction for cardiovascular events by application of the IL-1b specific antibody canakinumab, which subsequently lowered IL-6 and CRP levels. LDL-levels were not influenced. In patients with a high CRP reduction, a subsequent mortality reduction was shown. The LoDoCo trial showed a significantly (5.3% vs. 16%) lower rate of cardiovascular events over the time span of 3 years when patients received low-dose colchicine (0.5 mg/d) in addition to standard therapy [26]. The COLCOT trial [14] showed an analogous effect of colchicine on the secondary cardiovascular event rate in patients post-myocardial infarction. Colchicine inhibits IL-6 synthesis and, consecutively, lowers CRP plasma levels.

Of course, our short-term single-center observational study, in terms of quality, cannot be compared to these controlled randomized multi-center trials, but CRP is the common final stretch in all these trials and may, pathophysiologically, connect them.

Comparing cardiac glycosides to canakinumab, colchicine and recently described CRP apheresis [27–30], the following issues are crucial: 1. CRP apheresis is highly effective in acute disease, whereas it is likely that CRP synthesis inhibition is not; 2. Canakinumab and CRP apheresis are expensive therapies; 3. Canakinumab in CANTOS has shown immunosuppressive side effects, whereas CRP apheresis in CAMI-1 has not; and 4. Colchicine also is known to cause adverse events.

Thus, drugs with different mechanisms of action at lower costs would certainly reveal new horizons in the primary and secondary prevention of cardiovascular disease. Cardiac glycosides, however, do have a small therapeutic window with significant side effects outside the therapeutic range. Additionally, being $Na^{(+)}/K^{(+)}$-ATPase inhibitors, it may be a very long way to develop specific CRP synthesis inhibitors on the structural basis of cardiac glycosides. Consequently, these drugs can only theoretically be used as a pharmacological platform to develop agents that inhibit transcriptional CRP synthesis with less adverse event rates and, ideally, a wider therapeutic range in the distant future. The latter remains challenging.

4.4. Conclusions

The aim of C-DOS was to investigate whether digoxin is capable of lowering CRP levels in patients with heart failure and a left ventricular ejection fraction below 40%. A group comparison revealed borderline significance with a p-value of 0.051 (d21–d3), likely due to transcriptional CRP synthesis inhibition in vivo. C-DOS, although being a small and observational trial only, provides the first piece of evidence for CRP synthesis inhibition by cardiac glycosides in vivo in humans, and may be a "pilot study for subsequent phase III trials". A randomized controlled trial investigating the effect of cardiac glycosides on human CRP levels should be the next step, especially to exclude bystander effects. Cardiac glycosides may as well emerge as lead compounds for chemical modification in order to improve the potency, selectivity, and pharmacokinetics of CRP synthesis inhibition in cardiovascular disease.

Author Contributions: M.Z., K.K. and J.T. wrote the first draft, and conceptualized and finalized the manuscript. B.M., M.G. and O.Z. made substantial corrections. All authors have read and agreed to the published version of the manuscript.

Funding: This prospective observational cohort study was funded by the Hospital Association Allgaeug GmbH, Kempten, Germany.

Institutional Review Board Statement: The study was conducted in accordance with the Declaration of Helsinki, and approved by the Ethics Committee of the University of Ulm (protocol code: 28/12; date of approval: 8 February 2012) in 2012 and again in 2018 (protocol code: 28/12; date of approval: 22 October 2018) due to the reasons explained in detail in paragraph 2.1 of this manuscript.

Informed Consent Statement: Informed consent was obtained from all subjects involved in the study.

Data Availability Statement: Not applicable.

Conflicts of Interest: The authors declare no conflict of interest.

References

1. Pearson, T.A.; Mensah, G.A.; Alexander, R.W.; Anderson, J.L.; Cannon, R.O.; Criqui, M.; Fadl, Y.Y.; Fortmann, S.P.; Hong, Y.; Myers, G.L.; et al. Markers of inflammation and cardiovascular disease: Application to clinical and public health practice: A statement for healthcare professionals from the Centers for Disease Control and Prevention and the American Heart Association. *Circulation* **2003**, *107*, 499–511. [CrossRef] [PubMed]
2. Torzewski, J. C-reactive protein and atherogenesis: New insights from established animal models. *Am. J. Pathol.* **2005**, *167*, 923–925. [CrossRef]
3. Pepys, M.B. C-reactive protein is neither a marker nor a mediator of atherosclerosis. *Nat. Clin. Pract. Nephrol.* **2008**, *4*, 234–235. [CrossRef] [PubMed]
4. Reynolds, G.D.; Vance, R.P. C-reactive protein immunohistochemical localization in normal and atherosclerotic human aortas. *Arch. Pathol. Lab. Med.* **1987**, *111*, 265–269. [PubMed]
5. Torzewski, J.; Torzewski, M.; Bowyer, D.E.; Fröhlich, M.; Koenig, W.; Waltenberger, J.; Fitzsimmons, C.; Hombach, V. C-reactive protein frequently colocalizes with the terminal complement complex in the intima of early atherosclerotic lesions of human coronary arteries. *Arterioscler. Thromb. Vasc. Biol.* **1998**, *18*, 1386–1392. [CrossRef] [PubMed]
6. Yasojima, K.; Schwab, C.; McGeer, E.G.; McGeer, P.L. Generation of C-reactive protein and complement components in atherosclerotic plaques. *Am. J. Pathol.* **2001**, *158*, 1039–1051. [CrossRef]
7. Zacho, J.; Tybjaerg-Hansen, A.; Jensen, J.; Grande, P.; Sillesen, H.; Nordestgaard, B.G. Genetically elevated C-reactive protein and ischemic vascular disease. *N. Engl. J. Med.* **2008**, *30*, 1897–1908. [CrossRef] [PubMed]
8. Morita, H.; Nagai, R. Genetically elevated C-reactive protein and vascular disease. *N. Engl. J. Med.* **2009**, *360*, 934–935.
9. Taylor, K.E.; Giddings, J.C.; van den Berg, C.W. C-reactive protein-induced in vitro endothelial cell activation is an artefact caused by azide and lipopolysaccharide. *Arterioscler. Thromb. Vasc. Biol.* **2005**, *25*, 1225–1230. [CrossRef]
10. Kaplan, M.H.; Volanakis, J.E. Interaction of C-reactive protein complexes with the complement system. I. Consumption of human complement associated with the reaction of C-reactive protein with pneumococcal C-polysaccharide and with the choline phosphatides, lecithin and sphingomyelin. *J. Immunol.* **1974**, *112*, 2135–2147.
11. Bharadwaj, D.; Stein, M.P.; Volzer, M.; Mold, C.; Du Clos, T.W. The major receptor for C-reactive protein on leukocytes is fcgamma receptor II. *J. Exp. Med.* **1999**, *190*, 585–590. [CrossRef] [PubMed]
12. Ridker, P.M.; Danielson, E.; Fonseca, F.A.H.; Genest, J.; Gotto Jr, A.M.; Kastelein, J.J.P.; Koenig, W.; Libby, P.; Lorenzatti, A.J.; MacFadyen, J.G.; et al. JUPITER Study Group. Rosuvastatin to prevent vascular events in men and women with elevated C-reactive protein. *N. Engl. J. Med.* **2008**, *359*, 2195–2207. [CrossRef] [PubMed]
13. Ridker, P.M.; Everett, B.M.; Thuren, T.; MacFadyen, J.G.; Chang, W.H.; Ballantyne, C.; Fonseca, F.; Nicolau, J.; Koenig, W.; Anker, S.D.; et al. CANTOS Trial Group. Antiinflammatory Therapy with Canakinumab for atherosclerotic disease. *N. Engl. J. Med.* **2017**, *377*, 1119–1131. [CrossRef] [PubMed]
14. Tardif, J.C.; Kouz, S.; Waters, D.D.; Bertrand, O.F.; Diaz, R.; Maggioni, A.P.; Pinto, F.J.; Ibrahim, R.; Gamra, H.; Kiwan, G.S.; et al. Efficacy and Safety of Low-Dose Colchicine after Myocardial Infarction. *N. Engl. J. Med.* **2019**, *381*, 2497–2505. [CrossRef]
15. Kolkhof, P.; Geerts, A.; Schäfer, S.; Torzewski, J. Cardiac glycosides potently inhibit C-reactive protein synthesis in human hepatocytes. *Biochem. Biophys. Res. Commun.* **2010**, *394*, 233–239. [CrossRef]
16. Kostenzer, K. Anwendungsbeobachtung: Hemmung der Synthese des C-Reaktiven Proteins durch kardiale Glykoside. Ph.D. Thesis, Universität Ulm, Ulm, Germany, 2021. [CrossRef]
17. Torzewski, J.; Graf, M.; Weber, K.; Zaczkiewicz, M.; Leier, M.; Froehlich, M.; Zimmermann, O. Inhibiting C-Reactive Protein Synthesis by Cardiac Glycosides in Humans. *Open Conf. Proc. J.* **2016**, *7*, 7–11. [CrossRef]
18. Saylav, B.E.; Erdoğan, M.; Bahattin, Ö.; Ibrahim, S.; Ibrahim, S.; Canan, H.; Oytun, E. Short term protective effect of digitoxin in sepsis-induced acute lung injury. *Biocell* **2022**, *46*, 433–439. [CrossRef]
19. NVL Chronische Herzinsuffizienz, 3. Auflage. Available online: https://www.leitlinien.de/nvl/html/nvl-chronische-herzinsuffizienz/3-auflage/tabellenverzeichnis (accessed on 22 January 2022).
20. McMurray, J.J.; Adamopoulos, S.; Anker, S.D.; Auricchio, A.; Böhm, M.; Dickstein, K.; Falk, V.; Filippatos, G.; Fonseca, C.; Gomez-Sanchez, M.; et al. ESC Guidelines for the diagnosis and treatment of acute and chronic heart failure 2012: The Task Force for the Diagnosis and Treatment of Acute and Chronic Heart Failure 2012 of the European Society of Cardiology. Developed in collaboration with the Heart Failure Association (HFA) of the ESC. *Eur. Heart J.* **2012**, *33*, 17871847. [CrossRef]
21. Withering, W. *An Account of the Foxglove and Some of Its Medical Uses with Practical Remarks on Dropsy and Other Diseases*; GGJ and J Robinson: London, UK, 1785.
22. Yancy, C.W.; Jessup, M.; Bozkurt, B.; Butler, J.; Casey, D.E., Jr.; Colvin, M.M.; Drazner, M.H.; Filippatos, G.S.; Fonarow, G.C.; Givertz, M.M.; et al. ACC/AHA/HFSA Focused Update of the 2013 ACCF/AHA Guideline for the Management of Heart Failure: A Report of the American College of Cardiology/American Heart Association Task Force on Clinical Practice Guidelines and the Heart Failure Society of America. *Circulation* **2017**, *136*, e137–e161. [CrossRef]
23. Dávila, L.A.; Weber, K.; Bavendiek, U.; Bauersachs, J.; Wittes, J.; Yusuf, S.; Koch, A. Digoxin-mortality: Randomized vs. observational comparison in the DIG trial. *Eur. Heart J.* **2019**, *40*, 3336–3341. [CrossRef]

24. Andrade, J.; Khairy, P.; Dobrev, D.; Nattel, S. The clinical profile and pathophysiology of atrial fibrillation: Relationships among clinical features, epidemiology, and mechanisms. *Circ. Res.* **2014**, *114*, 145314–145368. [CrossRef] [PubMed]
25. Prasad, K. C-reactive (CRP)-lowering agents. *Cardiovasc. Drug Rev.* **2006**, *24*, 33–50. [CrossRef] [PubMed]
26. Nidorf, S.M.; Eikelboom, J.W.; Budgeon, C.A.; Thompson, P.L. Low-dose colchicine for secondary prevention of cardiovascular disease. *J. Am. Coll. Cardiol.* **2013**, *61*, 404–410. [CrossRef] [PubMed]
27. Sheriff, A.; Schindler, R.; Vogt, B.; Abdel-Aty, H.; Unger, J.K.; Bock, C.; Gebauer, F.; Slagman, A.; Jerichow, T.; Mans, D.; et al. Selective apheresis of C-reactive protein: A new therapeutic option in myocardial infarction? *J. Clin. Apher.* **2015**, *30*, 15–21. [CrossRef]
28. Ries, W.; Sheriff, A.; Heigl, F.; Zimmermann, O.; Garlichs, C.D.; Torzewski, J. "First in Man": Case Report of Selective C-Reactive Protein Apheresis in a Patient with Acute ST Segment Elevation Myocardial Infarction. *Case Rep. Cardiol.* **2018**, *2018*, 4767105. [CrossRef]
29. Ries, W.; Torzewski, J.; Heigl, F.; Pfluecke, C.; Kelle, S.; Darius, H.; Ince, H.; Mitzner, S.; Nordbeck, P.; Butter, C.; et al. C-Reactive Protein Apheresis as Anti-inflammatory Therapy in Acute Myocardial Infarction: Results of the CAMI-1 Study. *Front. Cardiovasc. Med.* **2021**, *8*, 155. [CrossRef]
30. Torzewski, J.; Heigl, F.; Zimmermann, O.; Wagner, F.; Schumann, C.; Hettich, R.; Bock, C.; Kayser, S.; Sheriff, A. First-in-Man: Case Report of Selective C-Reactive Protein Apheresis in a Patient with SARS-CoV-2 Infection. *Am. J. Case Rep.* **2020**, *21*, e925020. [CrossRef]

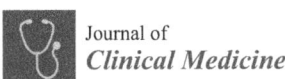

Article

Improved Prognostic Value in Predicting Long-Term Cardiovascular Events by a Combination of High-Sensitivity C-Reactive Protein and Brachial–Ankle Pulse Wave Velocity

Hack-Lyoung Kim *, Woo-Hyun Lim, Jae-Bin Seo, Sang-Hyun Kim, Joo-Hee Zo and Myung-A Kim

Boramae Medical Center, Division of Cardiology, Department of Internal Medicine, Seoul National University College of Medicine, 5 Boramae-ro, Dongjak-gu, Seoul 07061, Korea; woosion@gmail.com (W.-H.L.); cetuximab@naver.com (J.-B.S.); shkimmd@snu.ac.kr (S.-H.K.); jooheezo@hanmail.net (J.-H.Z.); kma@snu.ac.kr (M.-A.K.)
* Correspondence: khl2876@gmail.com; Tel.: +82-2-870-3235; Fax: +82-2-831-2826

Abstract: Background: Both C-reactive protein (CRP) and arterial stiffness are associated with the development of cardiovascular disease (CVD). This study was performed to investigate whether a combination of these two measurements could improve cardiovascular risk stratification. Methods: A total of 6572 consecutive subjects (mean age, 60.8 ± 11.8 years; female, 44.2%) who underwent both high-sensitivity CRP (hs-CRP) and brachial–ankle pulse wave velocity (baPWV) measurement within 1 week were retrospectively analyzed. Major adverse cardiovascular events (MACE), including cardiovascular death, acute myocardial infarction, coronary revascularization, and stroke were assessed during the clinical follow-up. Results: During a mean follow-up period of 3.75 years (interquartile range, 1.78–5.31 years), there were 182 cases of MACE (2.8%). The elevated baPWV ($\geq$1505 cm/s) (hazard ratio (HR), 4.21; 95% confidence interval (CI), 2.73–6.48; p < 0.001) and hs-CRP ($\geq$3 mg/L) (HR, 1.57; 95% CI, 1.12–2.21; p < 0.001) levels were associated with MACE even after controlling for potential confounders. The combination of baPWV and hs-CRP further stratified the subjects' risk (subjects with low baPWV and hs-CRP vs. subjects with high baPWV and hs-CRP; HR, 7.08; 95% CI, 3.76–13.30; p < 0.001). Adding baPWV information to clinical factors and hs-CRP had an incremental prognostic value (global Chi-square score, from 126 to 167, p < 0.001). Conclusions: The combination of hs-CRP and baPWV provided a better prediction of future CVD than either one by itself. Taking these two simple measurements simultaneously is clinically useful in cardiovascular risk stratification.

Keywords: arterial stiffness; C-reactive protein; major adverse cardiovascular event; pulse wave velocity; risk stratification

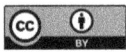

1. Introduction

Cardiovascular disease (CVD) is a leading cause of death and places a huge burden on our society worldwide [1]. Although various diagnostic and treatment methods have continuously been developed and applied to clinical practice, the prevalence of CVD is still high and the prognosis is poor. Identifying high-risk subjects who are more likely to develop CVD in the future and early implementation of active preventive strategies are critical to improving CVD prognosis [2]. While traditional risk factors represent cardiovascular risk well, they do not make all CVD incidences predictable [3]. In this respect, high-sensitivity C-reactive protein (hs-CRP), a sensitive marker for inflammation, has been recognized as a blood biomarker for predicting the occurrence of CVD. Inflammation plays a major role in the development and progression of atherosclerosis and the triggering of clinical CVD events [4]. Recent extensive evidence has suggested that high CRP levels are associated with higher risk of myocardial infarction, ischemic stroke, and sudden death [5–9].

Arteries stiffen with age and other risk factors, such as high blood pressure, hyperglycemia and smoking [10,11]. Of note, information on arterial stiffness is clinically valuable because it is associated with the occurrence of CVD, independent of traditional risk factors [12–19]. Of various methods of measuring arterial stiffness, pulse wave velocity (PWV) is most widely used in clinical and research fields [10].

Sometimes two test results are combined to improve the predictability of the prognosis [20,21]. Our group have also reported that PWV, along with noninvasive imaging studies, provides additional value in predicting the occurrence of CVD [22,23]. Although both hs-CRP and PWV have been used to predict CVD, there have been few studies on prognostic value by combining these two parameters. We hypothesized that the combination of hs-CRP and PWV would better predict the development of CVD. This study was performed to test this hypothesis.

2. Methods

2.1. Study Population

This single-center study was performed in a general hospital in a big city (Seoul, Korea). Between October 2008 and June 2018, a total of 8349 consecutive subjects who visited the cardiovascular center and underwent both brachial–ankle PWV (baPWV) and hs-CRP measurement within 1 week were retrospectively reviewed. The reasons for visiting the cardiovascular center vary widely, but it was not considered for study participation. The baPWV was measured by the attending physician as a routine part of a cardiovascular examination. Subjects with the following conditions were excluded from the study: (1) hs-CRP $\geq$ 10 mg/L (n = 1498) to rule out underlying active inflammatory conditions, (2) ankle-brachial index <0.9 or >1.4 (n = 85), (3) significant valvular dysfunction greater than mild degree (n = 43), (4) congenital heart disease (n = 6), (5) the presence of pericardial effusion (n = 12), and (6) atrial fibrillation and other uncontrolled arrhythmias (n = 133). Finally, 6572 subjects were analyzed in this study. This study was conducted in accordance with the declaration of Helsinki, revised in 2013. The study protocol was approved by the Institutional Review Board (IRB) of Boramae Medical Center (Seoul, Korea) and informed consent was waived due to the retrospective study design and the routine nature of information collected.

2.2. Data Collection

Body mass index was calculated as body weight in kilograms divided by the square of height in meters (kg/m^2). Obesity was defined as body mass index $\geq$25 kg/m^2. Hypertension was defined as previous diagnosis, current anti-hypertensive medications, or systolic and/or diastolic blood pressure $\geq$140/90 mmHg. Diabetes mellitus was defined as previous diagnosis, current anti-diabetic medications, or fasting blood glucose level $\geq$126 mg/dL. A person who smoked regularly in the last year was defined as a current smoker. Atherosclerotic cardiovascular disease (ASCVD) was defined as coronary artery disease including myocardial infarction and coronary revascularization, stroke, transient ischemic attack, and peripheral arterial disease [24]. After overnight fasting, blood samples were obtained in the antecubital vein and the blood levels of the following parameters were assessed: hemoglobin, creatinine, glucose, glycated hemoglobin, total cholesterol, low-density lipoprotein cholesterol, high-density lipoprotein cholesterol, triglyceride, and hs-CRP. Glomerular filtration rate was calculated by the Modification of Diet in Renal Disease (MDRD) study equation. Left ventricular ejection fraction was obtained by biplane Simpson's method on transthoracic echocardiography. Information on cardiovascular medications was obtained, which included calcium channel blocker, beta-blocker, renin-angiotensin system blocker, diuretic, and statin.

2.3. baPWV Measurement

On the day of baPWV measurement, subjects were banned from smoking, alcohol, and caffeine-containing beverages such as coffee or green tea. Usual medications were not stopped and continued to be taken. The subjects rested in bed for about 5 min before the examination. The measurements were taken in a quiet closed room with constant temperature and humidity. The baPWV measured using a VP-100 analyzer (Colins, Komaki, Japan) [23,25]. After wrapping blood pressure cuffs around both upper arms and ankles, pressure waveforms of the brachial and tibial arteries were recorded with plethysmographic and oscillometric pressure sensors using occlusion/sensing cuffs. The time intervals between pressure waveforms of the brachial and tibial arteries (pulse transit time) were measured, and baPWV was automatically calculated at the estimated distance from the patient's height [25]. The average of right and left baPWV measurements was used for analysis in this study. The baPWV was measured by an experienced operator. The coefficient of variation in baPWV measurement for intraobserver variability was 5.1% in our laboratory [26].

2.4. Clinical Events

The primary study endpoint, major adverse cardiovascular event (MACE), was composite clinical events consisting of cardiovascular death, non-fatal myocardial infarction, coronary revascularization, and stroke. Cardiovascular death included sudden cardiac death and death resulting from acute myocardial infarction, heart failure, stroke, cardiovascular procedures, cardiovascular hemorrhage, or other cardiovascular causes. Unexplained sudden death was considered cardiac death. Myocardial infarction was defined based on symptoms, electrocardiographic changes, elevation in cardiac troponin, and imaging results showing occlusive coronary artery lesions. Coronary revascularization included percutaneous coronary intervention and coronary bypass surgery. Stroke was diagnosed by neurologists using brain imaging study findings along with sudden neurological deficits.

2.5. Statistical Analysis

Continuous variables are expressed as mean ± standard deviation, and categorical variables are expressed as n (%). The means of continuous variables were compared using Student's t test, and the prevalences of categorical variables were compared using Chi-square test between the 2 groups. Multivariable cox regression analyses were performed to find independent associations of hs-CRP, baPWV, and their combination with MACE. Variables with statistical significance in univariable analyses were used as independent variables in multivariable analysis. Receiver operating characteristic (ROC) curve analysis was used to obtain the cut-off value of baPWV predicting MACE. For the analysis of hs-CRP-related MACE, subjects were stratified into 2 groups by CRP levels: <3 mg/L vs. ≥3 mg/L [27,28]. Kaplan–Meier survival curve analysis was used to show event-free survival rates according to hs-CRP, baPWV, and their combination values. The log-rank test was used to test statistical significance. Additional prognostic value of hs-CRP and baPWV was assessed using global Chi-square scores. A p value of <0.05 was considered statistically significant. All statistical analyses were performed using SPSS 22.0 (IBM Corp., Armonk, NY, USA).

3. Results

3.1. Baseline Clinical Characteristics of the Study Subjects

During a mean follow-up period of 3.75 years (interquartile range, 1.78–5.31 years), there were 182 cases of MACE (2.8%), which included 14 cardiac deaths, 19 myocardial infarction cases, 118 coronary revascularization cases, and 49 stroke cases. The baseline clinical characteristics of the study subjects are shown in Table 1. Subjects with MACE were older and it was more common in males. Subjects with MACE had more cardiovascular risk factors, including hypertension, diabetes mellitus, cigarette smoking, and history of ASCVD compared to those without MACE. In laboratory findings, subjects with MACE had lower levels of hemoglobin, glomerular filtration rate, total cholesterol, and left ventricular ejection fraction, as well as higher levels of glucose and glycated hemoglobin than those without. Cardiovascular medications including beta-blocker, renin-angiotensin system blocker, and statin were more frequently prescribed in subjects with MACE than those without. Both baPWV (1833 ± 378 cm/s vs. 1588 ± 340 cm, $p < 0.001$) and hs-CRP (3.26 ± 2.75 mg/L vs. 1.97 ± 2.31 mg/L, $p < 0.001$) were significantly higher in subjects with MACE than those without (Figure 1).

Table 1. Baseline clinical characteristics of study subjects.

Characteristic	Subjects with MACE (n = 182)	Subjects without MACE (n = 6390)	p
Age, years	64.7 ± 10.4	60.7 ± 11.8	<0.001
Male sex	123 (67.6)	3544 (55.5)	0.001
BMI, kg/m^2	24.8 ± 2.9	24.9 ± 3.3	0.626
Cardiovascular risk factors			
Hypertension	105 (57.7)	3102 (48.5)	0.015
Diabetes mellitus	56 (30.8)	1471 (23.0)	0.015
Obesity (BMI ≥ 25 kg/m^2)	79 (44.1)	2959 (46.4)	0.546
Cigarette smoking	49 (26.9)	1080 (16.9)	<0.001
Previous ASCVD	86 (43.7)	1470 (23.0)	<0.001
Laboratory findings			
Hemoglobin, g/dL	13.1 ± 2.0	13.6 ± 1.7	<0.001
GFR, mL/min/1.73m^2	82.7 ± 26.1	87.0 ± 23.7	0.016
Fasting glucose, mg/dL	129 ± 52	119 ± 39	0.012
Glycated hemoglobin, %	6.61 ± 1.21	6.27 ± 1.07	0.018
Total cholesterol, mg/dL	159 ± 44	165 ± 38	0.039
LDL cholesterol, mg/dL	93.9 ± 41.6	96.4 ± 35.4	0.428
HDL cholesterol, mg/dL	47.7 ± 15.4	49.2 ± 12.8	0.212
Triglyceride, mg/dL	131 ± 82	131 ± 84	0.964
LV ejection fraction, %	60.4 ± 10.1	63.6 ± 9.1	<0.001
Cardiovascular medications			
Calcium channel blocker	22 (12.1)	1094 (17.1)	0.075
Beta-blocker	69 (37.9)	1438 (22.5)	<0.001
RAS blocker	82 (45.1)	1990 (31.1)	<0.001
Statin	121 (66.5)	2915 (45.6)	<0.001

MACE, major adverse cardiovascular event; BMI, body mass index; ASCVD, atherosclerotic cardiovascular disease; GFR, glomerular filtration rate; LDL, low-density lipoprotein; HDL, high-density lipoprotein; LV, left ventricular; RAS, renin-angiotensin system.

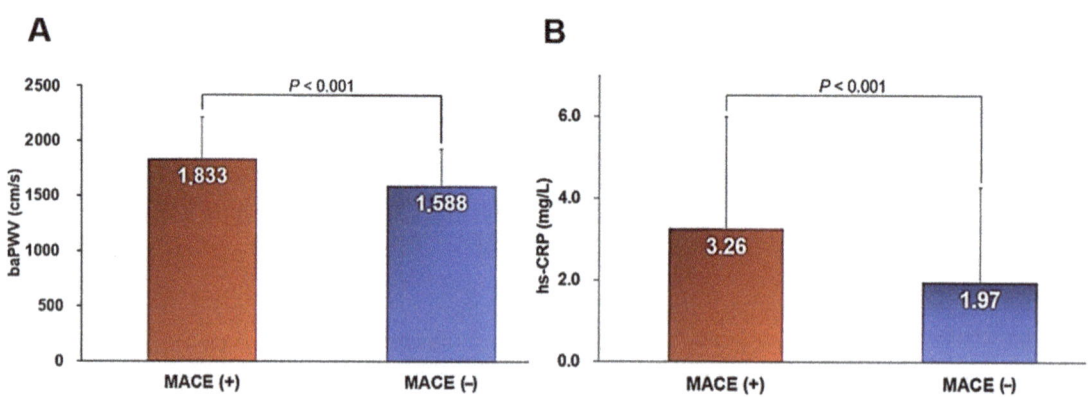

Figure 1. baPWV (A) and hs-CRP (B) values according to MACE. baPWV, brachial–ankle pulse wave velocity; hs-CRP, high-sensitivity C-reactive protein; MACE, major adverse cardiovascular events.

3.2. Associations of baPWV, hs-CRP, and Their Combinations with MACE

ROC curve analysis showed that a baPWV of 1505 cm/s was the cut-off value predicting MACE, with a sensitivity of 83.5% and a specificity of 46.0% (Figure 2). Multivariable analyses showing associations of hs-CRP, baPWV, and their combinations with MACE are shown in Table 2. The elevated hs-CRP (≥3 mg/L) (hazard ratio (HR), 1.57; 95% confidence interval (CI), 1.12−2.21; $p < 0.001$) and baPWV (≥1505 cm/s) (HR, 4.21; 95% CI, 2.73−6.48; $p < 0.001$) levels were associated with MACE even after controlling for potential confounders. The combination of hs-CRP and baPWV further stratified the subjects' risk (subjects with low hs-CRP and low baPWV vs. subjects with high hs-CRP and high baPWV; HR, 7.08; 95% CI, 3.76−13.30; $p < 0.001$). Kaplan–Meier survival curves demonstrated significant MACE differences according to hs-CRP (<3 mg/L vs. ≥3 mg/L, log-rank $p < 0.001$) and baPWV (<1505 cm/s vs. ≥1505 cm/s, log-rank $p < 0.001$) levels (Figure 3). In the Kaplan–Meier curve, by combining hs-CRP with baPWV, the subjects' risk was further subdivided (Figure 4). Another combination of the hs-CRP level (≥3 mg/L) and clinical variables (age; sex; hypertension; diabetes mellitus; cigarette smoking; previous history of atherosclerotic cardiovascular disease; hemoglobin; glomerular filtration rate; total cholesterol; left ventricular ejection fraction; and the use of beta-blocker, renin-angiotensin system blocker, and statin) significantly increased prognostic value in predicting MACE (global Chi-square score, from 108 to 126, $p < 0.001$). Furthermore, the combination of baPWV (≥1505 cm/s) and hs-CRP + clinical variables had an incremental prognostic value in predicting MACE (global Chi-square score, from 126 to 167, $p < 0.001$) (Figure 5).

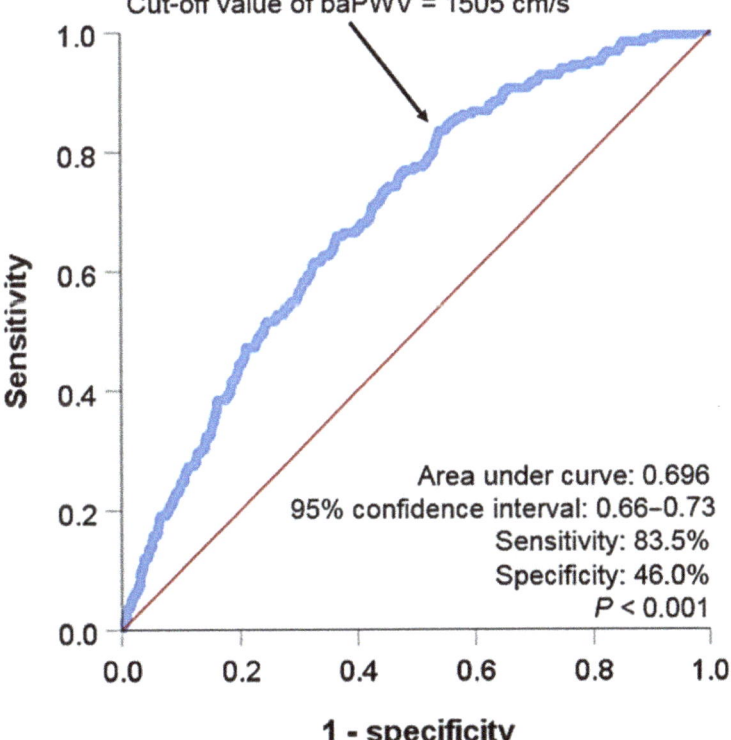

Figure 2. ROC curve analysis showing the cut-off value of baPWV for the MACE prediction. ROC, receiver operating characteristic; baPWV, brachial–ankle pulse wave velocity; MACE, major adverse cardiovascular events.

Table 2. Multivariable analyses showing the associations of baPWV, hs-CRP, and their combinations with MACE.

Variable	HR (95% CI)	p
hs-CRP ≥ 3 mg/L	1.57 (1.12−2.21)	<0.001
baPWV ≥ 1505 cm/s	4.21 (2.73−6.48)	<0.001
hs-CRP + baPWV		
hs-CRP < 3 mg/L and baPWV < 1505 cm/s	1	−
hs-CRP ≥ 3 mg/L and baPWV < 1505 cm/s	1.91 (0.89−4.10)	0.096
hs-CRP < 3 mg/L and baPWV ≥ 1505 cm/s	4.73 (2.57−8.70)	<0.001
hs-CRP ≥ 3 mg/L and baPWV ≥ 1505 cm/s	7.08 (3.76−13.30)	<0.001

Following clinical covariates were adjusted in each multivariable model: age; sex; hypertension; diabetes mellitus; cigarette smoking; previous history of atherosclerotic cardiovascular disease; hemoglobin, glomerular filtration rate; total cholesterol; left ventricular ejection fraction; and the use of beta-blocker, renin-angiotensin system blocker, and statin. baPWV, brachial–ankle pulse wave velocity; hs-CRP, high-sensitivity C-reactive protein; MACE, major adverse cardiovascular events; HR, hazard ratio; CI, confidence interval.

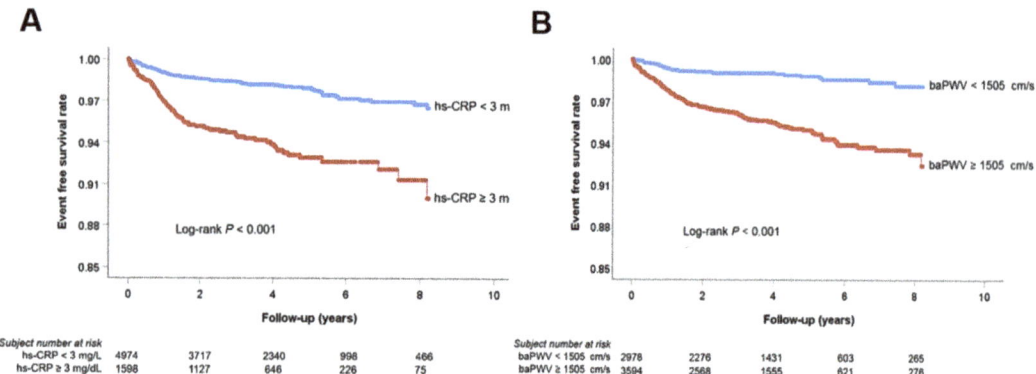

Figure 3. Kaplan–Meier survival curve analyses showing event-free survival rate according to hs-CRP (**A**) and baPWV (**B**). hs-CRP, high-sensitivity C-reactive protein; baPWV, brachial–ankle pulse wave velocity.

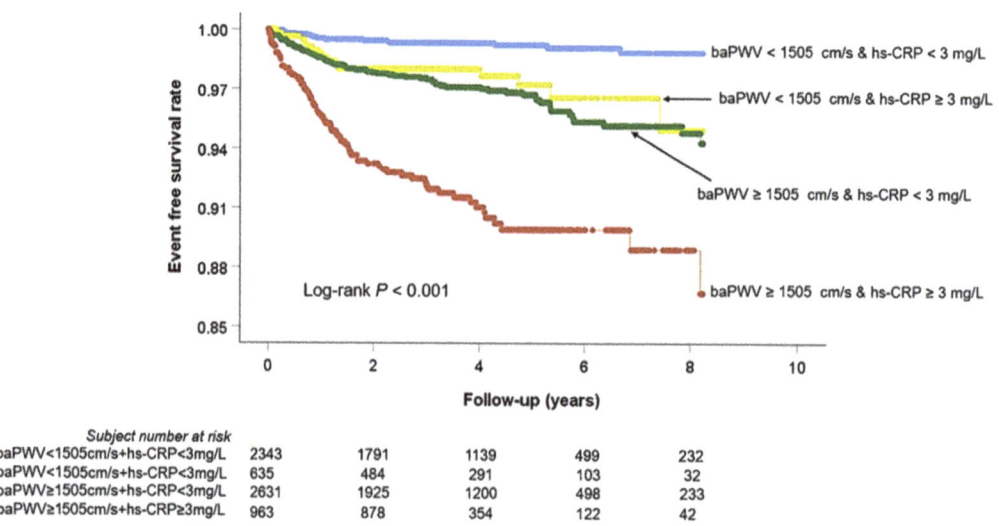

Figure 4. Kaplan–Meier survival curve analyses showing event free survival rate according to combination of hs-CRP and baPWV. hs-CRP, high-sensitivity C-reactive protein; baPWV, brachial-ankle pulse wave velocity.

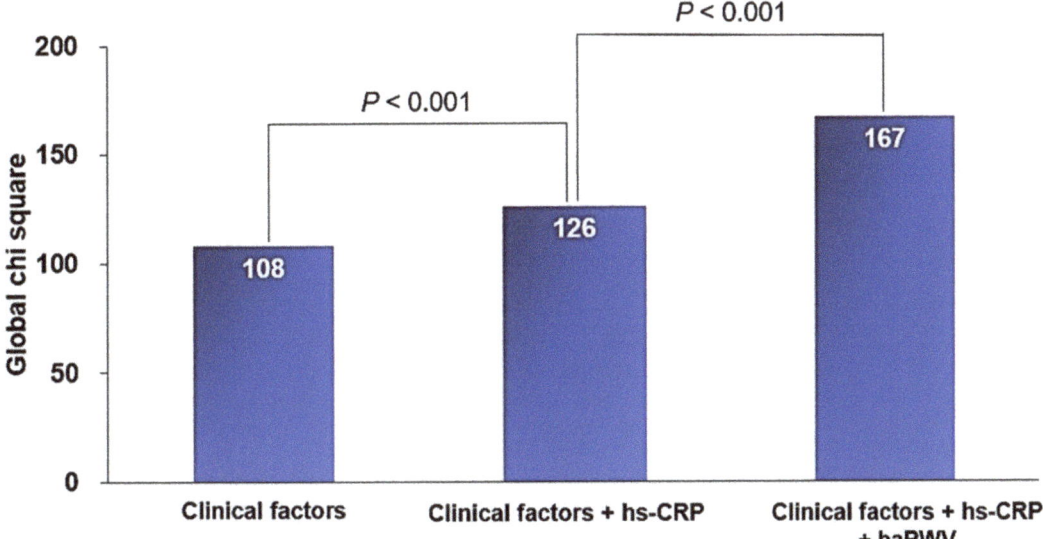

Figure 5. Incremental prognostic value of baPWV to clinical factors and hs-CRP. hs-CRP, high-sensitivity C-reactive protein; baPWV, brachial–ankle pulse wave velocity.

4. Discussion

Our results demonstrated that both increased hs-CRP and baPWV were independently associated with a higher risk for MACE in consecutive subjects visiting a cardiovascular center of a general hospital. More importantly, prognostic value was further improved by using a combination of hs-CRP and baPWV. Also, baPWV provided additional prognostic value in combination with clinical variables and hs-CRP in predicting MACE. To the best of our knowledge, this is the first study showing the improved prognostic value in predicting MACE by combining hs-CRP with baPWV.

4.1. Prognostic Value of CRP

CRP is a protein that increases synthesis in the liver against infection, inflammation, or tissue damage in our body. The level of CRP in the blood is proportional to the degree of synthesis in the liver [29]; thus, the blood level of CRP has been used for the diagnosis and treatment monitoring of infection or inflammatory disease. Due to the fact that the inflammatory response is deeply involved in the development and progression of atherosclerosis [4], CRP can also be a marker for atherosclerosis. In particular, inflammatory reactions in coronary plaques play an important role in plaque ruptures and subsequent acute atherothrombotic events [30]. There is also evidence that CRP is directly involved in the pathogenesis of atherothrombosis [31]. Many clinical studies have shown the association between elevated CRP and poor cardiovascular outcomes [5–9]. In line with these studies, our study also showed that baseline higher hs-CRP level (≥ 3 mg/L) was significantly associated with higher MACE incidences than those with lower hs-CRP level (<3 mg/L).

4.2. Prognostic Value of baPWV

Although carotid–femoral PWV (cfPWV) is the gold standard method for the non-invasive assessment of arterial stiffness [32], the clinical usefulness of baPWV, which is simpler to measure, is increasingly emerging [33,34]. The prognostic value of baPWV in predicting cardiovascular events has also been identified in many studies [13,17–19]. This study also showed that higher baPWV levels are independently associated with increased MACE incidences. The cut-off value of baPWV for predicting CVD has not yet been completely elucidated, and different cut-off values have been suggested in a different study population [18,35,36]. Therefore, we obtained the baPWV level that best predicts MACE in our study population through ROC curve analysis, and used it for survival analysis. It has been suggested that the cut-off value of baPWV that predicts future cardiovascular events depends on the subject's cardiovascular risk. In subjects with relatively low cardiovascular risk, such as the general public, the cut-off value of baPWV is around 1500 cm/s, and in high-risk patients, such as those with coronary artery disease or diabetes mellitus, the cut-off value of baPWV is 1700–1800 cm/s [34]. Since the subjects of this study were consecutive subjects visiting the cardiovascular center, the overall cardiovascular risk was not high, and may be similar to or slightly higher than the general population, so the proposed cut-off in our study of 1505 cm/s is similar to the results of previous studies.

4.3. Combination of hs-CRP and baPWV

The main concern of our study was whether the ability to predict cardiovascular risk increases when hs-CRP and baPWV information are combined. Several studies performed by our group have shown incremental prognostic value of baPWV when combined with other non-invasive tests [23,26]. In the present study, we showed that the combination of hs-CRP and baPWV more accurately predicted MACE occurrence, and adding baPWV information to hs-CRP and clinical factors significantly increased prognostic power. CRP measurement is inexpensive and can be easily performed using venous blood. The measurement of baPWV is also non-invasive and simple, and it is useful especially for mass screening [33,34]. Given our findings and the simplicity of hs-CRP and baPWV measurements, the combination of the two measurements seems cost-effective to predict cardiovascular risks.

4.4. Study Limitations

Besides its retrospective study design, our study has several limitations. First, it is possible that a selection bias has occurred because we assessed subjects who performed both baPWV and hs-CRP measurement within 1 week. Second, many clinical variables that appear to be associated with the subjects' cardiovascular risk were corrected in the multivariate analysis; however, we could not rule out the effects of possible uncorrected confounders. Lastly, our study population was restricted to Korean subjects, and generalization of our results to other ethnic groups is difficult.

5. Conclusions

Predicting cardiovascular risk is very important because early personalized treatment can improve a subject's prognosis. Both hs-CRP and baPWV are known to be good predictors of cardiovascular events. In this study, it was shown that the combination of hs-CRP and baPWV provided better prediction of future CVD than either one by itself. Given that both hs-CRP and baPWV tests are easy and inexpensive to measure, taking the two simple measurements simultaneously is clinically useful for better cardiovascular risk stratification.

Author Contributions: Formal analysis, H.-L.K.; Investigation, H.-L.K., W.-H.L., J.-B.S. and S.-H.K.; Methodology, W.-H.L. and M.-A.K.; Resources, W.-H.L., J.-B.S., S.-H.K., J.-H.Z. and M.-A.K.; Writing—original draft, H.-L.K.; Writing—review & editing, H.-L.K and J.-H.Z. All authors have read and agreed to the published version of the manuscript.

Funding: This research received no external funding.

Institutional Review Board Statement: The study was conducted according to the guidelines of the Declaration of Helsinki, and approved by the Institutional Review Board of Boramae Medical Center (IRB number, 10-2020-34 and date of approval, 17 April 2020).

Informed Consent Statement: Informed consent was waived due to the retrospective study design and the routine nature of information collected.

Conflicts of Interest: The authors declare no conflict of interest.

References

1. Virani, S.S.; Alonso, A.; Benjamin, E.J.; Bittencourt, M.S.; Callaway, C.W.; Carson, A.P.; Chamberlain, A.M.; Chang, A.R.; Cheng, S.; Delling, F.N.; et al. Heart Disease and Stroke Statistics-2020 Update: A Report from the American Heart Association. *Circulation* **2020**, *141*, e139–e596. [PubMed]
2. Arnett, D.K.; Blumenthal, R.S.; Albert, M.A.; Buroker, A.B.; Goldberger, Z.D.; Hahn, E.J.; Himmelfarb, C.D.; Khera, A.; Lloyd-Jones, D.; McEvoy, J.W.; et al. 2019 ACC/AHA Guideline on the Primary Prevention of Cardiovascular Disease: A Report of the American College of Cardiology/American Heart Association Task Force on Clinical Practice Guidelines. *Circulation* **2019**, *140*, e596–e646. [CrossRef]
3. Greenland, P.; Knoll, M.D.; Stamler, J.; Neaton, J.D.; Dyer, A.R.; Garside, D.B.; Wilson, P.W. Major risk factors as antecedents of fatal and nonfatal coronary heart disease events. *JAMA* **2003**, *290*, 891–897. [CrossRef] [PubMed]
4. Libby, P. Inflammation in atherosclerosis. *Nature* **2002**, *420*, 868–874. [CrossRef] [PubMed]
5. Koenig, W.; Sund, M.; Fröhlich, M.; Fischer, H.G.; Löwel, H.; Döring, A.; Hutchinson, W.L.; Pepys, M.B. C-Reactive protein, a sensitive marker of inflammation, predicts future risk of coronary heart disease in initially healthy middle-aged men: Results from the MONICA (Monitoring Trends and Determinants in Cardiovascular Disease) Augsburg Cohort Study. *Circulation* **1999**, *99*, 237–242. [CrossRef]
6. Wilson, P.W.F.; Nam, B.-H.; Pencina, M.; D'Agostino, R.B.; Benjamin, E.J.; O'Donnell, C.J. C-Reactive Protein and Risk of Cardiovascular Disease in Men and Women from the Framingham Heart Study. *Arch. Intern. Med.* **2005**, *165*, 2473–2478. [CrossRef]
7. Rost, N.S.; Wolf, P.A.; Kase, C.S.; Kelly-Hayes, M.; Silbershatz, H.; Massaro, J.; D'Agostino, R.B.; Franzblau, C.; Wilson, P.W. Plasma Concentration of C-Reactive Protein and Risk of Ischemic Stroke and Transient Ischemic Attack: The Framingham Study. *Stroke* **2001**, *32*, 2575–2579. [CrossRef]
8. He, L.-P.; Tang, X.-Y.; Ling, W.-H.; Chen, W.-Q.; Chen, Y.-M. Early C-reactive protein in the prediction of long-term outcomes after acute coronary syndromes: A meta-analysis of longitudinal studies. *Heart* **2010**, *96*, 339–346. [CrossRef]
9. Burke, A.P.; Tracy, R.P.; Kolodgie, F.; Malcom, G.T.; Zieske, A.; Kutys, R.; Pestaner, J.; Smialek, J.; Virmani, R. Elevated C-reactive protein values and atherosclerosis in sudden coronary death: Association with different pathologies. *Circulation* **2002**, *105*, 2019–2023. [CrossRef]
10. Cavalcante, J.L.; Lima, J.A.; Redheuil, A.; Al-Mallah, M.H. Aortic stiffness: Current understanding and future directions. *J. Am. Coll. Cardiol.* **2011**, *57*, 1511–1522. [CrossRef]
11. Lee, H.Y.; Oh, B.H. Aging and arterial stiffness. *Circ. J.* **2010**, *74*, 2257–2262. [CrossRef] [PubMed]
12. Vlachopoulos, C.; Aznaouridis, K.; Stefanadis, C. Prediction of Cardiovascular Events and All-Cause Mortality With Arterial Stiffness: A Systematic Review and Meta-Analysis. *J. Am. Coll. Cardiol.* **2010**, *55*, 1318–1327. [CrossRef]
13. Ohkuma, T.; Ninomiya, T.; Tomiyama, H.; Kario, K.; Hoshide, S.; Kita, Y.; Inoguchi, T.; Maeda, Y.; Kohara, K.; Tabara, Y.; et al. Brachial-ankle pulse wave velocity and the risk prediction of cardiovascular disease: An individual participant data meta-analysis. *Hypertension* **2017**, *69*, 1045–1052. [CrossRef] [PubMed]
14. Laurent, S.; Katsahian, S.; Fassot, C.; Tropeano, A.-I.; Gautier, I.; Laloux, B.; Boutouyrie, P. Aortic Stiffness Is an Independent Predictor of Fatal Stroke in Essential Hypertension. *Stroke* **2003**, *34*, 1203–1206. [CrossRef] [PubMed]
15. Sutton-Tyrrell, K.; Najjar, S.S.; Boudreau, R.; Venkitachalam, L.; Kupelian, V.; Simonsick, E.M.; Havlik, R.; Lakatta, E.G.; Spurgeon, H.; Kritchevsky, S.; et al. Elevated Aortic Pulse Wave Velocity, a Marker of Arterial Stiffness, Predicts Cardiovascular Events in Well-Functioning Older Adults. *Circulation* **2005**, *111*, 3384–3390. [CrossRef]
16. Hansen, T.; Staessen, J.A.; Torp-Pedersen, C.; Rasmussen, S.; Thijs, L.; Ibsen, H.; Jeppesen, J. Prognostic Value of Aortic Pulse Wave Velocity as Index of Arterial Stiffness in the General Population. *Circulation* **2006**, *113*, 664–670. [CrossRef]
17. Ahn, K.T.; Jeong, J.O.; Jin, S.A.; Kim, M.; Oh, J.K.; Choi, U.L.; Seong, S.W.; Kim, J.H.; Choi, S.W.; Jeong, H.S.; et al. Brachial-ankle PWV for predicting clinical outcomes in patients with acute stroke. *Blood Press* **2017**, *26*, 204–210. [CrossRef]
18. Kim, H.L.; Lim, W.H.; Seo, J.B.; Kim, S.H.; Zo, Z.H.; Kim, M.A. Prediction of cardiovascular events using brachial-ankle pulse wave ve-locity in hypertensive patients. *J. Clin. Hypertens* **2020**, *22*, 1659–1665. [CrossRef]
19. Meguro, T.; Nagatomo, Y.; Nagae, A.; Seki, C.; Kondou, N.; Shibata, M.; Oda, Y. Elevated Arterial Stiffness Evaluated by Brachial-Ankle Pulse Wave Velocity is Deleterious for the Prognosis of Patients with Heart Failure. *Circ. J.* **2009**, *73*, 673–680. [CrossRef]
20. Seo, W.-W.; Kim, H.-L.; Kim, Y.-J.; Yoon, Y.E.; Lee, S.-P.; Kim, H.-K.; Cho, G.-Y.; Zo, J.-H.; Choi, D.-J.; Sohn, D.-W. Incremental prognostic value of high-sensitive C-reactive protein in patients undergoing coronary computed tomography angiography. *J. Cardiol.* **2016**, *68*, 222–228. [CrossRef]
21. Liu, J.-H.; Chen, Y.; Yuen, M.; Zhen, Z.; Chan, C.W.-S.; Lam, K.S.-L.; Tse, H.-F.; Yiu, K.-H. Incremental prognostic value of global longitudinal strain in patients with type 2 diabetes mellitus. *Cardiovasc. Diabetol.* **2016**, *15*, 22. [CrossRef]
22. Jang, K.; Kim, H.-L.; Park, M.; Oh, S.; Oh, S.W.; Lim, W.-H.; Seo, J.-B.; Kim, S.-H.; Zo, J.-H.; Kim, M.-A. Additional Value of Brachial-Ankle Pulse Wave Velocity to Single-Photon Emission Computed Tomography in the Diagnosis of Coronary Artery Disease. *J. Atheroscler. Thromb.* **2017**, *24*, 1249–1257. [CrossRef] [PubMed]
23. Hwang, I.C.; Jin, K.N.; Kim, H.L.; Kim, Y.N.; Im, M.S.; Lim, W.H.; Seo, J.B.; Kim, S.H.; Zo, J.H.; Kim, M.A. Additional prognostic value of bra-chial-ankle pulse wave velocity to coronary computed tomography angiography in patients with suspected coronary artery disease. *Atherosclerosis* **2018**, *268*, 127–137. [CrossRef] [PubMed]

24. Grundy, S.M.; Stone, N.J.; Bailey, A.L.; Beam, C.; Birtcher, K.K.; Blumenthal, R.S. 2018 AHA/ACC/AACVPR/AAPA/ABC/ACPM/ADA/AGS/APhA/ASPC/NLA/PCNA Guideline on the Management of Blood Cholesterol: A Report of the American College of Cardiology/American Heart Association Task Force on Clinical Practice Guidelines. *J. Am. Coll. Cardiol.* **2019**, *73*, e285–e350. [CrossRef] [PubMed]
25. Yamashina, A.; Tomiyama, H.; Takeda, K.; Tsuda, H.; Arai, T.; Hirose, K.; Koji, Y.; Hori, S.; Yamamoto, Y. Validity, Reproducibility, and Clinical Significance of Noninvasive Brachial-Ankle Pulse Wave Velocity Measurement. *Hypertens. Res.* **2002**, *25*, 359–364. [CrossRef]
26. Lee, H.S.; Kim, H.L.; Kim, H.; Hwang, D.; Choi, H.M.; Oh, S.W.; Seo, J.B.; Chung, W.Y.; Kim, S.H.; Kim, M.A.; et al. Incremental prognostic value of brachial-ankle pulse wave velocity to single-photon emission computed tomography in patients with suspected cor-onary artery disease. *J. Atheroscler. Thromb.* **2015**, *22*, 1040–1050. [CrossRef]
27. Pearson, T.A.; Mensah, G.A.; Alexander, R.W.; Anderson, J.L.; Cannon, R.O., 3rd; Criqui, M.; Fadl, Y.Y.; Fortmann, S.P.; Hong, Y.; Myers, G.L.; et al. Markers of inflammation and cardiovascular disease: Application to clinical and public health practice: A statement for healthcare professionals from the Centers for Disease Control and Prevention and the American Heart Association. *Circulation* **2003**, *107*, 499–511. [CrossRef]
28. Mac Giollabhui, N.; Ellman, L.M.; Coe, C.L.; Byrne, M.L.; Abramson, L.Y.; Alloy, L.B. To exclude or not to exclude: Considerations and recommendations for C-reactive protein values higher than 10 mg/L. *Brain Behav. Immun.* **2020**, *87*, 898–900. [CrossRef] [PubMed]
29. Vigushin, D.M.; Pepys, M.B.; Hawkins, P.N. Metabolic and scintigraphic studies of radioiodinated human C-reactive protein in health and disease. *J. Clin. Investig.* **1993**, *91*, 1351–1357. [CrossRef] [PubMed]
30. Van der Wal, A.C.; Becker, A.E.; van der Loos, C.M.; Das, P.K. Site of intimal rupture or erosion of thrombosed coronary athero-sclerotic plaques is characterized by an inflammatory process irrespective of the dominant plaque morphology. *Circulation* **1994**, *89*, 36–44. [CrossRef]
31. Paffen, E.; DeMaat, M.P. C-reactive protein in atherosclerosis: A causal factor? *Cardiovasc Res.* **2006**, *71*, 30–39. [CrossRef] [PubMed]
32. Van Bortel, L.M.; Laurent, S.; Boutouyrie, P.; Chowienczyk, P.; Cruickshank, J.K.; De Backer, T.; Filipovsky, J.; Huybrechts, S.; Mattace-Raso, F.U.; Protogerou, A.D.; et al. Expert consensus document on the measurement of aortic stiffness in daily practice using carotid-femoral pulse wave velocity. *J. Hypertens.* **2012**, *30*, 445–448. [CrossRef] [PubMed]
33. Munakata, M. Brachial-ankle pulse wave velocity in the measurement of arterial stiffness: Recent evidence and clinical applications. *Curr. Hypertens. Rev.* **2014**, *10*, 49–57. [CrossRef] [PubMed]
34. Kim, H.L.; Kim, S.H. Pulse wave velocity in atherosclerosis. *Front. Cardiovasc. Med.* **2019**, *6*, 41. [CrossRef] [PubMed]
35. Kawai, T.; Ohishi, M.; Onishi, M.; Ito, N.; Takeya, Y.; Maekawa, Y.; Rakugi, H. Cut-off value of brachial-ankle pulse wave velocity to predict cardiovascular disease in hypertensive patients: A cohort study. *J. Atheroscler. Thromb.* **2013**, *20*, 391–400. [CrossRef] [PubMed]
36. Choi, J.-S.; Oh, S.J.; Sung, Y.W.; Moon, H.J.; Lee, J.S. Pulse wave velocity is a new predictor of acute kidney injury development after off-pump coronary artery bypass grafting. *PLoS ONE* **2020**, *15*, e0232377. [CrossRef]

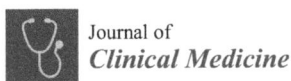

Review

The Complex Role of C-Reactive Protein in Systemic Lupus Erythematosus

Helena Enocsson [1], Jesper Karlsson [1], Hai-Yun Li [2], Yi Wu [2,3], Irving Kushner [4], Jonas Wetterö [1] and Christopher Sjöwall [1,*]

1. Department of Biomedical and Clinical Sciences, Division of Inflammation and Infection, Linköping University, SE-581 85 Linkoping, Sweden; helena.enocsson@liu.se (H.E.); jesper.karlsson@liu.se (J.K.); jonas.wettero@liu.se (J.W.)
2. MOE Key Laboratory of Environment and Genes Related to Diseases, School of Basic Medical Sciences, Xi'an Jiaotong University, West Yanta Road, Xi'an 710061, China; lihaiy@xjtu.edu.cn (H.-Y.L.); wuy@lzu.edu.cn (Y.W.)
3. The Affiliated Children's Hospital of Xi'an Jiaotong University, West Yanta Road, Xi'an 710061, China
4. Division of Rheumatology, Department of Medicine, Case Western Reserve University at MetroHealth Medical Center, 2500 MetroHealth Dr., Cleveland, OH 44109, USA; ixk2@case.edu
* Correspondence: christopher.sjowall@liu.se; Tel.: +46-10-1032416

Citation: Enocsson, H.; Karlsson, J.; Li, H.-Y.; Wu, Y.; Kushner, I.; Wetterö, J.; Sjöwall, C. The Complex Role of C-Reactive Protein in Systemic Lupus Erythematosus. *J. Clin. Med.* **2021**, *10*, 5837. https://doi.org/10.3390/jcm10245837

Academic Editors: Ahmed Sheriff and Emmanuel Andrès

Received: 10 November 2021
Accepted: 9 December 2021
Published: 13 December 2021

Publisher's Note: MDPI stays neutral with regard to jurisdictional claims in published maps and institutional affiliations.

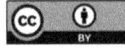

Copyright: © 2021 by the authors. Licensee MDPI, Basel, Switzerland. This article is an open access article distributed under the terms and conditions of the Creative Commons Attribution (CC BY) license (https://creativecommons.org/licenses/by/4.0/).

Abstract: C-reactive protein (CRP) is well-known as a sensitive albeit unspecific biomarker of inflammation. In most rheumatic conditions, the level of this evolutionarily highly conserved pattern recognition molecule conveys reliable information regarding the degree of ongoing inflammation, driven mainly by interleukin-6. However, the underlying causes of increased CRP levels are numerous, including both infections and malignancies. In addition, low to moderate increases in CRP predict subsequent cardiovascular events, often occurring years later, in patients with angina and in healthy individuals. However, autoimmune diseases characterized by the Type I interferon gene signature (e.g., systemic lupus erythematosus, primary Sjögren's syndrome and inflammatory myopathies) represent exceptions to the general rule that the concentrations of CRP correlate with the extent and severity of inflammation. In fact, adequate levels of CRP can be beneficial in autoimmune conditions, in that they contribute to efficient clearance of cell remnants and immune complexes through complement activation/modulation, opsonization and phagocytosis. Furthermore, emerging data indicate that CRP constitutes an autoantigen in systemic lupus erythematosus. At the same time, the increased risks of cardiovascular and cerebrovascular diseases in patients diagnosed with systemic lupus erythematosus and rheumatoid arthritis are well-established, with significant impacts on quality of life, accrual of organ damage, and premature mortality. This review describes CRP-mediated biological effects and the regulation of CRP release in relation to aspects of cardiovascular disease and mechanisms of autoimmunity, with particular focus on systemic lupus erythematosus.

Keywords: acute-phase protein; autoimmunity; cardiovascular risk; C-reactive protein; inflammation; organ damage; systemic lupus erythematosus

1. Introduction

Although more than 90 years have passed since the discovery of C-reactive protein (CRP) at The Rockefeller University, our current understanding of CRP is essentially based on the original observations made by William S. Tillett and Thomas Francis Jr. in the laboratory of Oswald T. Avery. They found that sera obtained from patients during the acute phase of pneumococcal pneumonia precipitated with the C-polysaccharide derived from the cell wall of the pneumococcus, and that this reaction diminished as the patients recovered [1,2]. This previously unknown C-reactive substance was later found to be a protein, and thus was named "C-reactive protein" [1,2]. The ligand to which CRP bound associated with teichoic acid and was identified in the 1970s as phosphorylcholine, which is abundant on the surfaces of microbes and apoptotic cells [3].

Today, we know that CRP is a highly conserved and ubiquitous protein in vertebrates and invertebrates [4]. In humans, CRP is a liver-derived acute-phase protein that consists of five identical 23-kDa globular subunits arranged in a pentameric structure with a discoid shape. In addition to the short pentraxins, CRP and serum amyloid P component (SAP), the pentraxin superfamily contains long pentraxins, i.e., neuronal pentraxin 1 (NPTX1), neuronal pentraxin 2 (NPTX2), neuronal pentraxin receptor (NPTXR), pentraxin 3 (PTX3), and pentraxin 4 (PTX4) [5].

The integrity of the native pentameric structure of CRP (pCRP) is dependent upon the presence of calcium ions. This structure is disrupted irreversibly into monomers under denaturing conditions, e.g., in an acidic microenvironment. Such CRP monomers (mCRP) appear to have distinct biological properties, which are often different from those of pCRP [6]. In addition, mCRP has been shown to act as an autoantigen in systemic lupus erythematosus (SLE), as well as in certain other diseases [7].

CRP is produced in large quantities by hepatocytes, mainly in response to the pro-inflammatory cytokine interleukin-6 (IL-6) [8]. The profound clinical interest in CRP arises from its use as a sensitive biomarker of ongoing bacterial infections, trauma, ischemic cardiovascular disease (CVD) and other inflammatory conditions, as well as its use as a crude discriminator of bacterial from viral infections, since bacterial infections typically yield higher levels of circulating CRP. However, in conditions characterized by the Type I interferon (IFN) gene signature (e.g., SLE, primary Sjögren's syndrome and inflammatory myopathies), CRP appears to be an unreliable marker of inflammation, since the circulating levels of CRP can be modest—despite the presence of extensive inflammation, as evidenced by an increased level of IL-6 in the circulation [9,10]. Furthermore, several studies of cardiovascular and autoimmune diseases have highlighted the importance of the genetic regulation of CRP [11,12].

In parallel with the discovery that a low-level increase in CRP is a useful risk marker for cardiovascular events, substantial progress has been made over the last decades concerning the biological properties and physiological importance of CRP in both health and disease. This review summarizes recent discoveries related to CRP-mediated biological effects, as well as to the regulation of CRP release with respect to aspects of CVD and mechanisms of autoimmunity.

2. CRP as a Biomarker in Rheumatologic Diseases

CRP is the main biomarker of inflammation used in modern healthcare. In most laboratories in Europe, for routine detection of CRP, the cut-off defining an abnormal level is set at 5 or 10 mg/L. However, for estimation of CVD risk, a 'high-sensitivity' CRP assay is usually applied [13,14]. At Linköping University Hospital (Sweden), the lower limit of quantification for this high-sensitivity CRP assay is 0.15 mg/L.

Historically, CRP has not always been the most popular biomarker reflecting inflammation. Several other acute-phase proteins show different concentration pattern changes in the plasma over time; some of these increase (e.g., serum amyloid A) and some decrease (e.g., albumin) during the acute-phase response [15,16]. In rheumatology, the erythrocyte sedimentation rate (ESR), which is a reflector of ongoing inflammation, deserves special attention. However, whereas the kinetics of ESR is slightly different from that of CRP, it conveys different information and can be affected by various factors, such as the erythrocyte count and fibrinogen and immunoglobulin concentrations.

In the newest set of classification criteria for rheumatoid arthritis (RA), 'abnormal CRP and/or ESR' is regarded as a separate item together with joint involvement, presence of autoantibodies and duration of symptoms [17]. CRP levels >10 mg/L are frequently seen in untreated patients with recent-onset RA. Other types of arthritis show different tendencies to display abnormal CRP levels. During an attack of gout, the concentration of CRP can become impressively high, often arousing a suspicion of septic arthritis. In spondylo-arthritides, such as psoriatic arthritis (PsoA), high CRP levels are usually less common, although patients with involvement of large joints may constitute exceptions to this. Consequently, abnormal levels of acute-phase proteins were not included in the classification criteria for PsoA [18].

In giant cell arteritis (GCA), unexplained high levels of CRP and ESR, accompanied by unspecific symptoms such as weight-loss and headache, may lead to a correct diagnosis [19]. GCA may present with or without proximal muscular pain, referred to as polymyalgia rheumatica (PMR). Besides muscular involvement, the 2012 classification criteria for PMR require both age ≥ 50 years and abnormal CRP and/or ESR levels [20]. In cases of anti-neutrophil cytoplasm antibody (ANCA)-associated vasculitis, high levels of CRP elevation are almost ubiquitous and appear to be associated with a higher risk of renal involvement [21].

While CRP levels usually parallel disease activity in inflammatory states, it is widely accepted that CRP is an unreliable biomarker in active SLE. Still, substantial CRP responses are observed in subsets of patients with SLE with certain manifestations (e.g., serositis and polyarthritis) [10,22]. In similarity to trivial viral infections, wherein the CRP levels typically remain low, SLE may manifest as oral ulcers, pleuritis/pericarditis and leukopenia, all of which commonly affect patients with viral infections. Another feature shared by viral infections and systemic inflammatory conditions, such as SLE, primary Sjögren's syndrome and inflammatory myopathies, is the activation of the Type I interferon system [23,24]. This will be discussed in depth below (Section 5).

Although CRP is a valuable biomarker in the clinical management of several rheumatic conditions, it must always be interpreted with caution and in the context of the symptoms presented by the patient. Several of the immunosuppressive agents used in rheumatology render the patients more prone to infections; this is particularly true for high doses of corticosteroids [25]. The risks for malignancies and paraneoplastic syndromes, which mimic rheumatic diseases, are important to consider, especially as the risks for certain cancers are increased in patients with rheumatic diseases [26,27]. Finally, some of the immunosuppressive drugs in use today directly affect the ability of the hepatocytes to produce adequate levels of CRP. The most obvious examples of this are the IL-6 receptor inhibitors tocilizumab and sarilumab, which are mainly used in cases of RA, systemic juvenile idiopathic arthritis and GCA [28]. Moreover, IL-6 signaling (and consequently CRP) may also be significantly negatively affected in patients who are receiving Janus kinase inhibitors and high doses of corticosteroids.

3. CRP as a Biomarker Indicating Increased Risks of Cerebrovascular and Cardiovascular Diseases

Based on the results of several prospective epidemiologic studies, CRP has emerged as one of the most powerful predictors of CVD in the general population [29]. In the 'Fragmin during Instability in Coronary Artery Disease' (FRISC) trial, which included almost 1000 patients with unstable coronary artery disease, the CRP levels were strongly associated with long-term risk of death from cardiac causes, independently of other established risk factors (i.e., hypertension, smoking, diabetes, dyslipidemia) [14]. Furthermore, CRP has been shown to contribute to several stages of atherogenesis, such as endothelial dysfunction, atherosclerotic plaque formation, plaque maturation, and plaque destabilization and eventual rupture [30].

Patients with RA, as well as those with SLE, have increased mortality compared to the general population [31,32]. Increased mortality from CVD has been reported in epidemiologic studies that have focused on RA [33]. In similarity to RA, the risk of CVD-related death is increased in SLE [31,34].

In prospective studies, the incidence rates of myocardial infarction and stroke in patients with SLE have been found to be high. The relative risk of myocardial infarction or stroke compared to the normal population is approximately 2–3 [35–37]. The highest relative risks have been reported for premenopausal women (8–50-fold higher risk), early in the course of SLE (<1 year after diagnosis, risk increased 4–10-fold), and in patients with renal involvement (4–18-fold higher risk) [38–40]. Other studies have focused on examining the incidence of CVD in patients with SLE compared to the expected CVD incidence, based on the presence of traditional risk factors. Even here, the incidence of CVD has been found to be considerably higher than expected [41,42]. In addition, risk of mortality post-myocardial infarction seems to be higher in patients with SLE than in the normal population, at least in the short term, while the long-term risk of mortality post-stroke is also increased [43,44].

Approximately 30% of patients with SLE display antiphospholipid antibodies (at least one of the following: anticardiolipin or anti-β2-glycoprotein-I antibodies, or a positive lupus anticoagulant test) and about 15–20% suffer from antiphospholipid syndrome (APS), which is characterized by an increased risk of thromboembolic disease and/or pregnancy morbidity. Ischemic stroke is the most common arterial manifestation of APS, while myocardial infarction is less common [45].

Whereas some studies have focused on CRP levels as a risk factor for future cardiovascular events in RA, studies of CRP levels in patients with SLE in relation to risks of CVD or stroke are scarce [46–49]. Statin therapy is likely to be safe and seems to result in significant reduction of plasma CRP concentrations in patients with SLE [50]. For patients with SLE, the Systemic Lupus International Collaborating Clinics/American College of Rheumatology (SLICC/ACR) Damage Index (SDI) constitutes a validated instrument to assess irreversible organ damage, including myocardial infarction and stroke [51]. We identified two studies in which CRP levels were analyzed in relation to accrual of damage. In the Hopkins Lupus cohort, Lee et al. showed that serum CRP levels (measured with the high-sensitivity technique) were independently associated with the total SDI score, although not specifically for myocardial infarction or stroke [52]. Our group has reported a similar association between CRP and global SDI [53]. Furthermore, in the SLICC cohort, we evaluated whether CRP could be predictive in terms of future damage accrual but obtained negative results [54].

4. Immunoregulatory Functions of CRP and other Pentraxins in SLE

The high accumulation of apoptotic cell debris and the formation of antinuclear antibodies (ANA), together with dysfunctional elimination of immune complexes are all key features of SLE pathogenesis [55]. In this context, it is of particular interest that CRP immune function can be viewed as a less specific albeit rapidly produced innate ancestor version of the phylogenetically more recent antibodies of adaptive immunity [56]. CRP is a pattern-recognition molecule of the innate immune system, and its binding to ligands such as surface-exposed phosphorylcholine on, for example, cellular debris can mediate direct prophagocytotic opsonization [57] and interactions with immunoglobulin receptors (Fc receptors) [56], as well as trigger 'classical' complement activation [58]. The latter promotes additional opsonization through subsequent covalent surface-binding of activated complement proteins.

Immune complex clearance is generally supported by efficient classical complement activation, and SLE pathogenesis is indeed intimately related to this activation pathway. Although homozygous complement deficiencies are extremely rare, they tell us a great deal about the normal physiological activities of the complement system in humans [59]. Homozygous genetic deficiencies in the initial proteins of the classical complement pathway (C1 proteins) are linked to a very high risk of developing SLE [60], and single nucleotide polymorphisms of the *CRP* gene are associated with ANA formation and SLE, possibly via the lowering of CRP levels [12].

In vertebrates, surface binding via the recognition face of the CRP molecule activates the calcium-dependent classical arm of the complement cascade by binding complement protein 1q (C1q) via its effector face [61,62]. C1q binding to the mCRP isoform has been demonstrated [63], and mCRP is capable of supporting complement-dependent phagocytosis and the oxidative burst in phagocytes [64]. Unlike immunoglobulin G-triggered classical activation, CRP-mediated initiation of the classical route typically does not proceed to the membrane-attack complex-forming 'terminal' stage of complement activation [65]. This is most likely due to direct interactions of CRP with inhibitory complement regulators.

It is well-established that CRP can bind to the soluble complement inhibitor factor H without compromising its inhibitory function, thereby limiting the continued activation of complement via the convertases, by accelerating their decay [66–69] and by serving as co-factor for Factor I in cleaving surface-bound C3b [70,71]. In addition, surface-bound mCRP can bind Factor H and, thereby, modulate complement activation [72]. Anti-C1q autoantibodies are frequently detected in lupus nephritis (LN) [73,74] and it is possible that autoantibodies targeting other proteins linked to classical complement activation, e.g., CRP, could affect the complement-mediated clearance of cellular debris [75,76]. CRP (and/or PTX3), complement, and immunoglobulins may co-localize with electron-dense deposits in glomerular LN [77,78]. Furthermore, it is possible that pre-immunization with pentraxins, leading to the triggering of anti-PTX3 antibody development, prevents progression to LN [77]. Anti-CRP antibodies appear to target mainly the motifs of mCRP (further described in Section 7) and are typically associated with LN. The mCRP amino acids 35–47 have been reported to represent an autoantibody target motif that is especially prone to anti-CRP binding in LN. From the complement-immunomodulatory point-of-view, it is interesting to note that this epitope also facilitates factor H binding and activity—which could be reversed by anti-CRP antibodies [79]. In accordance with this, factor H levels are low in LN and factor H dysregulation and polymorphisms are associated with active nephritis [80,81]. Other members of the factor H family, i.e., factor H-related Proteins 1 and 5, have recently been shown to be capable of binding DNA and subsequently recruiting mCRP and enhancing complement activation [82]. In addition, factor H-related Protein 4 has been reported to bind pCRP [83,84].

Ligand-bound CRP on necrotic cells and/or otherwise immobilized CRP can recruit the classical pathway inhibitor C4-binding protein (C4bp) while retaining the complement-inhibitory activity of C4bp [85,86]. It is possible that this C4bp–CRP interaction limits CRP–C1q binding [85,86], and thereby subsequent classical activation. Classical complement activation triggered by ligand-bound CRP may be downregulated during substantial increases in the concentrations of CRP, presumably through humoral CRP–C1q consumption [63,87]. This could also be of pathophysiologic relevance in SLE, where the CRP levels can be low despite active inflammation. Related to the now well-established role of collectins in the 'lectin' activation pathway of complement, a potential role of CRP in conveying C1q-dependent complement activation by collectin Placenta 1 has been reported [88]. This is a topic that would be interesting to pursue further in relation to autoimmune diseases.

In similarity to IgG, surface-bound CRP (and other pentraxins) can bind directly to all Fcγ-receptors [89], potentially activating phagocytes and facilitating elimination via phagocytosis, which is highly relevant for waste disposal mechanisms. The low-affinity FcγRIIa (CD32) has emerged as the primary functional CRP receptor [56,89–91]. However, unlike IgG, the CRP–FcγRIIa interaction depends on the R allele of the receptor polymorphism at amino acid 131 [92]. Since SLE pathogenesis is linked to immune complex-induced production of IFN-α by plasmacytoid dendritic cells, it is highly interesting to note that FcγRIIa also mediates the initial internalization of immune complexes that prompts intracellular TLR activation and activation of IFN-α [93]. Considering the protective effects of CRP seen in animal models of lupus, it is tempting to speculate that CRP acts as a modulator of IFN-α production by altering the immune complex handling by plasmacytoid dendritic cells. Accordingly, Mold and Du Clos reported that CRP indeed inhibits such immune complex-triggered activation of IFN-α, although the mechanism appeared to involve instead the endosomal processing of immune complexes [94]. Additional mechanistic studies on the CRP-mediated downregulation of immune complex-triggered IFN-α in SLE are highly warranted. Another intriguing finding that merits further attention is the potentially immunomodulatory effect of the CRP interaction with FcαRI, the IgA receptor [95].

5. Regulation of CRP Synthesis in SLE

Hepatocytes are considered the major source of CRP, although extrahepatic syntheses have been reported [96–100]. The *CRP* gene is located on chromosome 1q23.2 and hepatic production of CRP is mainly regulated at the transcriptional level, with IL-6 and IL-1β being the most important inducers [101,102]. IL-6 signaling in hepatocytes mediates the activation and CRP promoter-binding of signal inducer and activator of transcription 3 (STAT3) [102] and the CCAAT/enhancer binding protein β (C/EBPβ) [101,103]. In hepatic cell lines, the addition of IL-1β and subsequent NF-κB activation are usually required for *CRP* transcription, whereas in primary hepatocytes, IL-6 is sufficient for CRP production [101,104,105].

Although CRP is generally an excellent biomarker of inflammation and tissue damage due to its massive increase in level upon IL-6 induction, it is not useful in all inflammatory conditions. SLE represents an exception, in that the CRP levels rarely mirror the disease activity [15,106]. Inflammatory myopathies, primary Sjögren's syndrome and systemic sclerosis are other diseases for which CRP is considered an unreliable marker for monitoring disease activity [107]. In addition, viral infections rarely exhibit a substantial rise in CRP levels [108].

The above-mentioned conditions all have in common the activation of Type I IFNs. The most widely studied Type I IFN is IFN-α, which comprises 12 subtypes. Apart from having a physiologic function in defense against viruses, IFN-α induces and maintains autoimmune pathology through facilitation of autoantibody production and many other functions, as reviewed elsewhere [109]. Receptors for Type I IFNs (IFN-α/β receptor; IFNAR) are ubiquitously expressed and mediate the activation of different STAT heterodimers and homodimers for the activation of antiviral, inflammatory and regulatory gene expression [110]. Already in 2008, Type I IFNs were highlighted as potential inhibitors of CRP production via their activation of STAT1, so as to counteract the STAT3 effects, and/or the activation of an inhibitory isoform of C/EBPβ [10]. Later, an inhibitory effect of IFN-α (all subtypes) on CRP transcription and production was indeed shown in a hepatic cell line and in primary hepatocytes, respectively [104]. Further in vivo studies of CRP levels and IFN-α levels in patients with SLE have lent support to the notion of a regulatory role for IFN-α in CRP production [54,111], although the exact intracellular pathways remain unknown.

Polymorphisms of the *CRP* gene have been linked to differences in basal CRP levels and the risk of SLE and/or cardiovascular events [12,112–114]. One of these polymorphisms, rs1205, has been studied together with IL-6 and IFN-α with respect to the impact of these potential regulators of CRP levels in SLE, revealing lower CRP levels in patients with IFNα activation and/or the CRP-lowering polymorphism rs1205 (Figure 1). Thus, the relative lack of CRP response seen in viral infections and Type I IFN-driven autoimmune diseases can be attributed to an IFN-α-dependent downregulation of CRP transcription, as well as *CRP* gene polymorphisms, which are over-represented among patients with SLE [111,115].

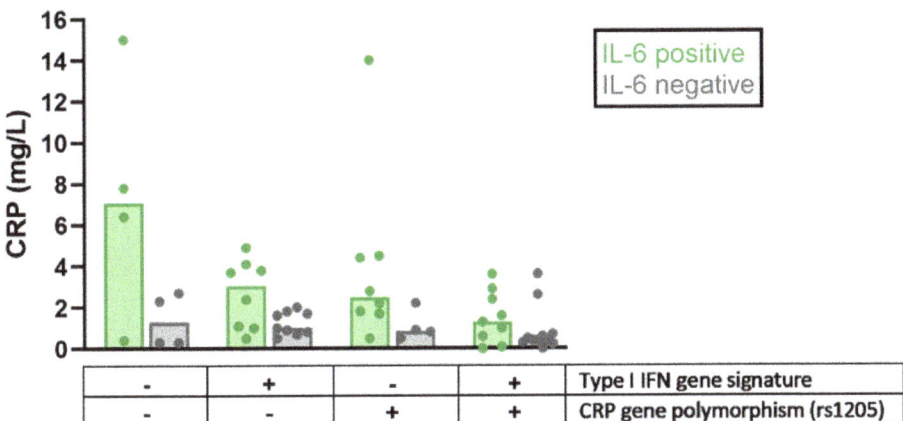

Figure 1. Differences in C-reactive protein (CRP) levels among patients with systemic lupus erythematosus (SLE) stratified based on the presence of detectable interleukin 6 (IL-6) levels, Type I interferon (IFN) gene signature, and CRP-lowering gene polymorphism (rs1205), respectively. All patients had a low disease activity but could be serologically active at sampling. Bars indicate median values. Dots represent individual values. Data shown in the figure were adopted from Enocsson et al. [115], with permission from Frontiers Media, 2021 (Creative Commons Attribution licence, version 4.0).

6. Structural Isoforms of CRP with Distinctive Biologic Effects

As mentioned above, pCRP can under certain conditions dissociate irreversibly into the monomeric form (mCRP), which displays distinctly different conformational characteristics and antigenic epitopes [116,117]. Emerging data implicate mCRP as the main CRP isoform that regulates local inflammatory processes [118–120]. Furthermore, mCRP may bind to IgG-containing immune complexes and facilitate silent Fc receptor-mediated removal via the reticuloendothelial system and complement deficiencies may result immune complex deposition outside the reticuloendothelial system [121,122].

Cell death occurs during inflammation, and the damaged cell membrane in apoptosis or necrosis is the main target of CRP recognition [4]. Using electron microscopy, the detection of new epitopes of the antigen, and immunofluorescence colocalization, Ji et al. have shown that the binding of CRP to the damaged cell membrane induces rapid transformation to mCRP, and that this dissociation process is accompanied by significant enhancement of complement activation and cellular stimulation capacity [118]. Eisenhardt et al. obtained similar results with activated platelet membranes [123]. In addition, inflammatory conditions such as moderate acidification and oxidative stress also promote conformational switching from pCRP to mCRP.

During acute inflammatory cardiovascular events, such as thrombosis and myocardial infarction, the CRP levels increase rapidly, while activated platelets in blood vessels or cell necrosis caused by hypoxia in the heart provide abundant damaged membrane ligands for CRP dissociation, which leads to the accumulation of a large amount of 'active' mCRP in the lesions within a short period of time [118,124]. This results in the excessive activation of neutrophils, platelets, monocytes and complement, thereby exacerbating the inflammation [118,123,125–130]. Furthermore, the conversion of pCRP to mCRP has been observed on microparticles in the blood obtained from patients who suffered myocardial infarctions, as well as on beta-amyloid plaques [131,132]. This process indicates a physiologic mechanism of CRP isomerization that is driven by the inflammatory microenvironment and, at the same time, supports the concept of mCRP occurring as a natural isomer of CRP and being involved in regulating inflammatory processes [120,133].

Most of the abovementioned dissociation scenarios for generating mCRP are specifically linked to inflammation. Thus, it is plausible that mCRP is generated predominately within the inflamed local tissue. Based on the strong proinflammatory activities of mCRP, we propose that, in addition to being an activating mechanism, the conversion of pCRP to mCRP serves as a buffering mechanism that localizes the proinflammatory actions to the site of the inflammation [118]. This mechanism could protect the body from systemic challenge in response to increased circulating levels of pCRP. It is worth noting that the bioactivities of mCRP largely overlap with, and occasionally exceed, those previously ascribed to pCRP. These bioactivities of mCRP include the activation of complement and the stimulation of endothelial cells, neutrophils and platelets, as well as its binding to ligands, e.g., LDL, C1q and factor H [63,72,85,126,128,134–143]. This raises the possibility that some of the reported actions of pCRP originate from mCRP formed during the purification process and/or storage.

The allosteric switch from pCRP, as a marker of inflammation, to functional mCRP that actually participates in the inflammatory process, enables this acute-phase protein to play active roles in a controlled manner under different pathophysiologic conditions. Thus, CRP can be regarded as a potential fine tuner of inflammation. Although there have been long-term debates about the biological significance of mCRP, recent studies have revealed the pathway of mCRP production, the regulatory effects of mCRP on innate and adaptive humoral immunity and inflammatory processes, and the presence of mCRP in focal tissues [63,118,123,126,128,134–138,142,144,145].

Interfering with the dissociation of CRP and the way in which mCRP exerts its biologic functions are candidate pathways towards designing treatment strategies for CVD. Since the specific contribution of mCRP depends on the inflammatory microenvironment, a clear understanding of the molecular mechanisms that act in different pathophysiologic conditions is a prerequisite for the design and selection of appropriate interventions. Several important issues remain to be resolved: (1) how to establish either direct or indirect detection methods that use mCRP as a disease marker; (2) how to establish an association between mCRP and disease processes; (3) how to describe the short-and long-term response profiles of different cell types to mCRP in a systematic way; and (4) identification of the receptor (s) that mediate the downstream effects of mCRP in lipid rafts.

7. Autoantibodies Directed against CRP in SLE and Related Conditions

Already in the mid-1980s, the presence of autoantibodies against CRP was described and linked to the debilitated ability of CRP to solubilize chromatin in a patient with SLE [146]. Subsequently, Bell et al. reported a high frequency of IgG antibodies to cryptic epitopes of CRP, first in patients suffering from the 'autoimmune-like' toxic oil syndrome and thereafter in patients with SLE [147,148]. Similarly, we have shown a prevalence of anti-CRP antibodies of approximately 40% in patients with SLE, with a distinct positive correlation between antibody occurrence/concentration and disease activity.

In our first study, we demonstrated that some patients with SLE were anti-CRP antibody positive on one occasion but negative on another occasion [149]. In succeeding investigations, we analyzed the antibody levels in consecutive samples from 10 well-characterized patients with SLE and showed that the levels of anti-CRP antibodies paralleled the clinical disease activity, usually with high levels of these antibodies appearing during disease flares [150]. In total, 70% of the patients were positive for anti-CRP antibodies on at least one occasion, and the levels correlated with disease activity assessed using the SLE disease activity index (SLEDAI).

Our findings were essentially confirmed by Rosenau and Schur, who demonstrated the presence of antibodies against CRP in the sera obtained from patients with different rheumatologic conditions, including SLE, where they observed an autoantibody frequency of 23% [151]. However, in our hands, sera from patients with RA or inflammatory bowel disease have consistently been negative in the anti-CRP assay, whereas a few additional patients with primary Sjögren's syndrome and chronic hepatitis C infection tested positive [149,152]. Others have found anti-CRP antibodies in patients with tubulointerstitial nephritis and uveitis (TINU) syndrome [153]. Furthermore, Figueredo et al. have demonstrated the presence of anti-CRP antibodies in patients with SLE with or without APS;

the anti-CRP-positive cases with SLE had lower C3 levels and were more likely to have anti-dsDNA and anticardiolipin antibodies as compared to the anti-CRP antibody-negative individuals. In addition, the frequency of LN was higher among the anti-CRP antibody positive SLE cases [154]. The biological properties of anti-CRP antibodies have also been investigated. Janko et al. demonstrated that anti-CRP—as well as anti-dsDNA-antibodies bind to apoptotic materials and, via clearance by macrophages, induce a pro-inflammatory cytokine response [75].

More recently, a large longitudinal study from Europe identified the presence of anti-CRP antibodies at the onset of LN as a strong risk factor for a composite outcome of non-response, renal flare, and end-stage renal disease after 2 years of standard LN treatment [155]. Analyses of the antigen specificity of the anti-CRP assay have revealed that autoantibodies to CRP in SLE are directed towards hidden epitopes, or neo-epitopes, of CRP (e.g., mCRP), and that immune complexes isolated from SLE sera do not induce false positive anti-CRP antibody test results [79,156,157]. Thus, in similarity to anti-C1q antibodies in SLE, reacting exclusively with an epitope that is exposed on structurally modified C1q [59,158], anti-CRP antibodies bind to mCRP on cells, as well as on tissues and in solution [76].

8. Conclusions

Even though almost a century has passed since the discovery of CRP, the biological effects of this highly conserved molecule are still poorly understood. Nonetheless, emerging data highlight the importance of structural isoforms of CRP and their associations with the complement system and CVD. As summarized in Figure 2, CRP plays a complex role in SLE—a disease in which CRP, in contrast to most other rheumatic conditions, constitutes an unreliable biomarker of inflammation. Recent data indicate that the combined effects of genetics and the Type I IFN signature are responsible for the dissociated correlation between CRP and IL-6 levels in patients with SLE. Given the potential activities of CRP in facilitating the removal of apoptotic debris and immune complexes, this may be of high relevance in terms of driving LN and the accrual of organ damage in SLE.

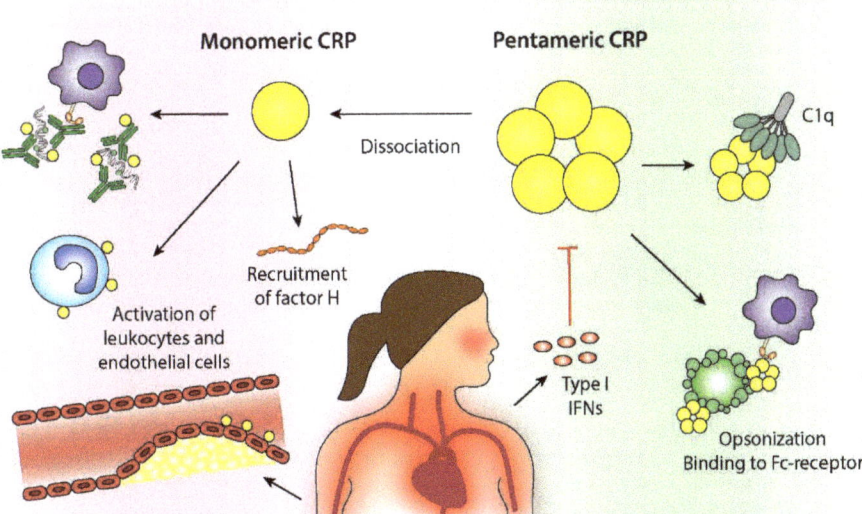

Figure 2. Immunoregulatory effects of pentameric C-reactive protein (pCRP) and monomeric CRP (mCRP) in the context of systemic lupus erythematosus (SLE) and cardiovascular disease. Dissociation of pCRP to mCRP will take place in inflammatory conditions and at cell surfaces and results in local immunoregulatory effects. The biological properties of mCRP partly overlaps the pCRP effects but is generally ascribed a more active and proinflammatory profile. CRP binds to and opsonizes dying cells and cell remnants, which facilitates phagocytosis via Fc-receptor binding. Furthermore, CRP activates classical complement activation via its binding to C1q, resulting in increased opsonization by C3b. Recruitment of

Factor H will however limit progression of the complement cascade to membrane attack complex formation. Increased levels of CRP can therefore contribute to efficient clearance of potential autoantigens and thus, be beneficial in autoimmune conditions. The ability of CRP to facilitate immune complex elimination further implies a protective role of CRP in autoimmune diseases. However, increased Type I IFN activity, frequently observed in patients with SLE, inhibits CRP production, which theoretically could increase the autoantigen burden and disease activity. Proatherogenic and prothrombotic effects of CRP are attributed to its stimulation of endothelial cells, neutrophils and platelets.

Author Contributions: Conceptualization, C.S.; search strategy and review of publications, H.E., J.K., H.-Y.L., Y.W., J.W. and C.S.; draft preparation, review and editing, H.E., J.K., H.-Y.L., Y.W., I.K., J.W. and C.S. All authors have read and agreed to the published version of the manuscript.

Funding: This work was supported by grants from Region Östergötland (ALF Grants), the Swedish Rheumatism Association, the Ulla and Roland Gustafsson Foundation, the King Gustaf V's 80-year Anniversary foundation and the King Gustaf V and Queen Victoria's Freemasons foundation.

Institutional Review Board Statement: Not applicable.

Informed Consent Statement: Not applicable.

Acknowledgments: The authors thank Lina Wirestam for the schematic illustration (Figure 2).

Conflicts of Interest: The authors declare no conflict of interest.

References

1. Tillett, W.S.; Francis, T. Serological Reactions in Pneumonia with a Non-Protein Somatic Fraction of Pneumococcus. *J. Exp. Med.* **1930**, *52*, 561–571. [CrossRef]
2. Kushner, I.; Samols, D. Oswald Avery and the pneumococcus. *Pharos Alpha Omega Alpha Honor Med. Soc.* **2011**, *74*, 14–18.
3. Volanakis, J.E.; Kaplan, M.H. Specificity of C-reactive protein for choline phosphate residues of pneumococcal C-polysaccharide. *Proc. Soc. Exp. Biol. Med.* **1971**, *136*, 612–614. [CrossRef] [PubMed]
4. Pepys, M.B.; Hirschfield, G.M. C-reactive protein: A critical update. *J. Clin. Invest.* **2003**, *111*, 1805–1812. [CrossRef] [PubMed]
5. Wang, Z.; Wang, X.; Zou, H.; Dai, Z.; Feng, S.; Zhang, M.; Xiao, G.; Liu, Z.; Cheng, Q. The Basic Characteristics of the Pentraxin Family and Their Functions in Tumor Progression. *Front Immunol.* **2020**, *11*, 1757. [CrossRef] [PubMed]
6. Wu, Y.; Potempa, L.A.; El Kebir, D.; Filep, J.G. C-reactive protein and inflammation: Conformational changes affect function. *Biol. Chem.* **2015**, *396*, 1181–1197. [CrossRef] [PubMed]
7. Brilland, B.; Vinatier, E.; Subra, J.F.; Jeannin, P.; Augusto, J.F.; Delneste, Y. Anti-Pentraxin Antibodies in Autoimmune Diseases: Bystanders or Pathophysiological Actors? *Front Immunol.* **2021**, *11*, 626343. [CrossRef]
8. Black, S.; Kushner, I.; Samols, D. C-reactive Protein. *J. Biol. Chem.* **2004**, *279*, 48487–48490. [CrossRef]
9. Gabay, C.; Roux-Lombard, P.; de Moerloose, P.; Dayer, J.M.; Vischer, T.; Guerne, P.A. Absence of correlation between interleukin 6 and C-reactive protein blood levels in systemic lupus erythematosus compared with rheumatoid arthritis. *J. Rheumatol.* **1993**, *20*, 815–821.
10. Gaitonde, S.; Samols, D.; Kushner, I. C-reactive protein and systemic lupus erythematosus. *Arthritis. Rheum.* **2008**, *59*, 1814–1820. [CrossRef]
11. Kuhlenbaeumer, G.; Huge, A.; Berger, K.; Kessler, C.; Voelzke, H.; Funke, H.; Stoegbauer, F.; Stoll, M.; Ringelstein, E.B. Genetic variants in the C-reactive protein gene are associated with microangiopathic ischemic stroke. *Cerebrovasc Dis.* **2010**, *30*, 476–482. [CrossRef] [PubMed]
12. Russell, A.I.; Cunninghame Graham, D.S.; Shepherd, C.; Roberton, C.A.; Whittaker, J.; Meeks, J.; Powell, R.J.; Isenberg, D.A.; Walport, M.J.; Vyse, T.J. Polymorphism at the C-reactive protein locus influences gene expression and predisposes to systemic lupus erythematosus. *Hum. Mol. Genet.* **2004**, *13*, 137–147. [CrossRef] [PubMed]
13. Antonelli, M.; Kushner, I. It's time to redefine inflammation. *FASEB J.* **2017**, *31*, 1787–1791. [CrossRef]
14. Lindahl, B.; Toss, H.; Siegbahn, A.; Venge, P.; Wallentin, L. Markers of myocardial damage and inflammation in relation to long-term mortality in unstable coronary artery disease. FRISC Study Group. Fragmin during Instability in Coronary Artery Disease. *N. Engl. J. Med.* **2000**, *343*, 1139–1147. [CrossRef]
15. Gabay, C.; Kushner, I. Acute-phase proteins and other systemic responses to inflammation. *N. Engl. J. Med.* **1999**, *340*, 448–454. [CrossRef] [PubMed]
16. Wirestam, L.; Pihl, S.; Saleh, M.; Wetterö, J.; Sjöwall, C. Plasma C-Reactive Protein and Pentraxin-3 Reference Intervals During Normal Pregnancy. *Front. Immunol.* **2021**, *12*, 722118. [CrossRef]
17. Aletaha, D.; Neogi, T.; Silman, A.J.; Funovits, J.; Felson, D.T.; Bingham, C.O., 3rd; Birnbaum, N.S.; Burmester, G.R.; Bykerk, V.P.; Cohen, M.D.; et al. 2010 rheumatoid arthritis classification criteria: An American College of Rheumatology/European League Against Rheumatism collaborative initiative. *Ann. Rheum. Dis.* **2010**, *69*, 1580–1588. [CrossRef] [PubMed]

18. Taylor, W.; Gladman, D.; Helliwell, P.; Marchesoni, A.; Mease, P.; Mielants, H.; Group, C.S. Classification criteria for psoriatic arthritis: Development of new criteria from a large international study. *Arthritis. Rheum.* **2006**, *54*, 2665–2673. [CrossRef] [PubMed]
19. Hellmich, B.; Agueda, A.; Monti, S.; Buttgereit, F.; de Boysson, H.; Brouwer, E.; Cassie, R.; Cid, M.C.; Dasgupta, B.; Dejaco, C.; et al. 2018 Update of the EULAR recommendations for the management of large vessel vasculitis. *Ann. Rheum. Dis.* **2020**, *79*, 19–30. [CrossRef] [PubMed]
20. Dasgupta, B.; Cimmino, M.A.; Kremers, H.M.; Schmidt, W.A.; Schirmer, M.; Salvarani, C.; Bachta, A.; Dejaco, C.; Duftner, C.; Jensen, H.S.; et al. 2012 Provisional classification criteria for polymyalgia rheumatica: A European League Against Rheumatism/American College of Rheumatology collaborative initiative. *Arthritis. Rheum.* **2012**, *64*, 943–954. [CrossRef] [PubMed]
21. Kronbichler, A.; Shin, J.I.; Lee, K.H.; Nakagomi, D.; Quintana, L.F.; Busch, M.; Craven, A.; Luqmani, R.A.; Merkel, P.A.; Mayer, G.; et al. Clinical associations of renal involvement in ANCA-associated vasculitis. *Autoimmun. Rev.* **2020**, *19*, 102495. [CrossRef] [PubMed]
22. Morrow, W.J.; Isenberg, D.A.; Parry, H.F.; Snaith, M.L. C-reactive protein in sera from patients with systemic lupus erythematosus. *J. Rheumatol.* **1981**, *8*, 599–604. [PubMed]
23. Bianchi, M.; Kozyrev, S.V.; Notarnicola, A.; Hultin Rosenberg, L.; Karlsson, M.; Pucholt, P.; Rothwell, S.; Alexsson, A.; Sandling, J.K.; Andersson, H.; et al. Contribution of rare genetic variation to disease susceptibility in a large Scandinavian myositis cohort. *Arthritis. Rheumatol.* **2021**. Epub Ahead of Print. [CrossRef] [PubMed]
24. Imgenberg-Kreuz, J.; Almlof, J.C.; Leonard, D.; Sjöwall, C.; Syvanen, A.C.; Rönnblom, L.; Sandling, J.K.; Nordmark, G. Shared and Unique Patterns of DNA Methylation in Systemic Lupus Erythematosus and Primary Sjogren's Syndrome. *Front Immunol.* **2019**, *10*, 1686. [CrossRef] [PubMed]
25. Strangfeld, A.; Eveslage, M.; Schneider, M.; Bergerhausen, H.J.; Klopsch, T.; Zink, A.; Listing, J. Treatment benefit or survival of the fittest: What drives the time-dependent decrease in serious infection rates under TNF inhibition and what does this imply for the individual patient? *Ann. Rheum. Dis.* **2011**, *70*, 1914–1920. [CrossRef]
26. Askling, J. Malignancy and rheumatoid arthritis. *Curr. Rheumatol. Rep.* **2007**, *9*, 421–426. [CrossRef]
27. Manger, B.; Schett, G. Paraneoplastic syndromes in rheumatology. *Nat. Rev. Rheumatol.* **2014**, *10*, 662–670. [CrossRef]
28. Ogata, A.; Kato, Y.; Higa, S.; Yoshizaki, K. IL-6 inhibitor for the treatment of rheumatoid arthritis: A comprehensive review. *Mod. Rheumatol.* **2019**, *29*, 258–267. [CrossRef] [PubMed]
29. Ridker, P.M.; Hennekens, C.H.; Buring, J.E.; Rifai, N. C-reactive protein and other markers of inflammation in the prediction of cardiovascular disease in women. *N. Engl. J. Med.* **2000**, *342*, 836–843. [CrossRef]
30. de Ferranti, S.D.; Rifai, N. C-reactive protein: A nontraditional serum marker of cardiovascular risk. *Cardiovasc. Pathol.* **2007**, *16*, 14–21. [CrossRef]
31. Bernatsky, S.; Boivin, J.F.; Joseph, L.; Manzi, S.; Ginzler, E.; Gladman, D.D.; Urowitz, M.; Fortin, P.R.; Petri, M.; Barr, S.; et al. Mortality in systemic lupus erythematosus. *Arthritis. Rheum.* **2006**, *54*, 2550–2557. [CrossRef] [PubMed]
32. Sparks, J.A.; Chang, S.C.; Liao, K.P.; Lu, B.; Fine, A.R.; Solomon, D.H.; Costenbader, K.H.; Karlson, E.W. Rheumatoid Arthritis and Mortality Among Women During 36 Years of Prospective Follow-Up: Results From the Nurses' Health Study. *Arthritis. Care Res.* **2016**, *68*, 753–762. [CrossRef]
33. Avina-Zubieta, J.A.; Choi, H.K.; Sadatsafavi, M.; Etminan, M.; Esdaile, J.M.; Lacaille, D. Risk of cardiovascular mortality in patients with rheumatoid arthritis: A meta-analysis of observational studies. *Arthritis. Rheum.* **2008**, *59*, 1690–1697. [CrossRef]
34. Björnadal, L.; Yin, L.; Granath, F.; Klareskog, L.; Ekbom, A. Cardiovascular disease a hazard despite improved prognosis in patients with systemic lupus erythematosus: Results from a Swedish population based study 1964-95. *J. Rheumatol.* **2004**, *31*, 713–719. [PubMed]
35. Arkema, E.V.; Svenungsson, E.; Von Euler, M.; Sjöwall, C.; Simard, J.F. Stroke in systemic lupus erythematosus: A Swedish population-based cohort study. *Ann. Rheum. Dis.* **2017**, *76*, 1544–1549. [CrossRef]
36. Avina-Zubieta, J.A.; To, F.; Vostretsova, K.; De Vera, M.; Sayre, E.C.; Esdaile, J.M. Risk of Myocardial Infarction and Stroke in Newly Diagnosed Systemic Lupus Erythematosus: A General Population-Based Study. *Arthritis. Care Res.* **2017**, *69*, 849–856. [CrossRef] [PubMed]
37. Samuelsson, I.; Parodis, I.; Gunnarsson, I.; Zickert, A.; Hofman-Bang, C.; Wallen, H.; Svenungsson, E. Myocardial infarctions, subtypes and coronary atherosclerosis in SLE: A case-control study. *Lupus. Sci. Med.* **2021**, *8*, e000515. [CrossRef] [PubMed]
38. Bengtsson, C.; Ohman, M.L.; Nived, O.; Rantapaa Dahlqvist, S. Cardiovascular event in systemic lupus erythematosus in northern Sweden: Ancidence and predictors in a 7-year follow-up study. *Lupus* **2012**, *21*, 452–459. [CrossRef]
39. Hermansen, M.L.; Lindhardsen, J.; Torp-Pedersen, C.; Faurschou, M.; Jacobsen, S. The risk of cardiovascular morbidity and cardiovascular mortality in systemic lupus erythematosus and lupus nephritis: A Danish nationwide population-based cohort study. *Rheumatology* **2017**, *56*, 709–715. [CrossRef] [PubMed]
40. Manzi, S.; Meilahn, E.N.; Rairie, J.E.; Conte, C.G.; Medsger, T.A., Jr.; Jansen-McWilliams, L.; D'Agostino, R.B.; Kuller, L.H. Age-specific incidence rates of myocardial infarction and angina in women with systemic lupus erythematosus: Comparison with the Framingham Study. *Am. J. Epidemiol.* **1997**, *145*, 408–415. [CrossRef]
41. Esdaile, J.M.; Abrahamowicz, M.; Grodzicky, T.; Li, Y.; Panaritis, C.; du Berger, R.; Cote, R.; Grover, S.A.; Fortin, P.R.; Clarke, A.E.; et al. Traditional Framingham risk factors fail to fully account for accelerated atherosclerosis in systemic lupus erythematosus. *Arthritis. Rheum.* **2001**, *44*, 2331–2337. [CrossRef]

42. Fischer, L.M.; Schlienger, R.G.; Matter, C.; Jick, H.; Meier, C.R. Effect of rheumatoid arthritis or systemic lupus erythematosus on the risk of first-time acute myocardial infarction. *Am. J. Cardiol.* **2004**, *93*, 198–200. [CrossRef] [PubMed]
43. Ke, S.R.; Liu, C.W.; Wu, Y.W.; Lai, K.R.; Wu, C.Y.; Lin, J.W.; Chan, C.L.; Pan, R.H. Systemic lupus erythematosus is associated with poor outcome after acute myocardial infarction. *Nutr. Metab. Cardiovasc. Dis.* **2019**, *29*, 1400–1407. [CrossRef]
44. Rossides, M.; Simard, J.F.; Svenungsson, E.; von Euler, M.; Arkema, E.V. Mortality and Functionality after Stroke in Patients with Systemic Lupus Erythematosus. *J. Rheumatol.* **2017**, *44*, 1590–1596. [CrossRef]
45. Svenungsson, E.; Antovic, A. The antiphospholipid syndrome - often overlooked cause of vascular occlusions? *J. Intern. Med.* **2020**, *287*, 349–372. [CrossRef]
46. Goodson, N.J.; Symmons, D.P.; Scott, D.G.; Bunn, D.; Lunt, M.; Silman, A.J. Baseline levels of C-reactive protein and prediction of death from cardiovascular disease in patients with inflammatory polyarthritis: A ten-year followup study of a primary care-based inception cohort. *Arthritis. Rheum.* **2005**, *52*, 2293–2299. [CrossRef] [PubMed]
47. Innala, L.; Möller, B.; Ljung, L.; Magnusson, S.; Smedby, T.; Södergren, A.; Ohman, M.L.; Rantapaa-Dahlqvist, S.; Wallberg-Jonsson, S. Cardiovascular events in early RA are a result of inflammatory burden and traditional risk factors: A five year prospective study. *Arthritis Res. Ther.* **2011**, *13*, R131. [CrossRef] [PubMed]
48. Maradit-Kremers, H.; Nicola, P.J.; Crowson, C.S.; Ballman, K.V.; Gabriel, S.E. Cardiovascular death in rheumatoid arthritis: A population-based study. *Arthritis. Rheum.* **2005**, *52*, 722–732. [CrossRef]
49. Kao, A.H.; Wasko, M.C.; Krishnaswami, S.; Wagner, J.; Edmundowicz, D.; Shaw, P.; Cunningham, A.L.; Danchenko, N.; Sutton-Tyrrell, K.; Tracy, R.P.; et al. C-reactive protein and coronary artery calcium in asymptomatic women with systemic lupus erythematosus or rheumatoid arthritis. *Am. J. Cardiol.* **2008**, *102*, 755–760. [CrossRef]
50. Sahebkar, A.; Rathouska, J.; Derosa, G.; Maffioli, P.; Nachtigal, P. Statin impact on disease activity and C-reactive protein concentrations in systemic lupus erythematosus patients: A systematic review and meta-analysis of controlled trials. *Autoimmun. Rev.* **2016**, *15*, 344–353. [CrossRef]
51. Gladman, D.; Ginzler, E.; Goldsmith, C.; Fortin, P.; Liang, M.; Urowitz, M.; Bacon, P.; Bombardieri, S.; Hanly, J.; Hay, E.; et al. The development and initial validation of the Systemic Lupus International Collaborating Clinics/American College of Rheumatology damage index for systemic lupus erythematosus. *Arthritis. Rheum.* **1996**, *39*, 363–369. [CrossRef] [PubMed]
52. Lee, S.S.; Singh, S.; Link, K.; Petri, M. High-sensitivity C-reactive protein as an associate of clinical subsets and organ damage in systemic lupus erythematosus. *Semin. Arthritis. Rheum.* **2008**, *38*, 41–54. [CrossRef]
53. Enocsson, H.; Wetterö, J.; Skogh, T.; Sjöwall, C. Soluble urokinase plasminogen activator receptor levels reflect organ damage in systemic lupus erythematosus. *Transl. Res.* **2013**, *162*, 287–296. [CrossRef] [PubMed]
54. Enocsson, H.; Wirestam, L.; Dahle, C.; Padyukov, L.; Jonsen, A.; Urowitz, M.B.; Gladman, D.D.; Romero-Diaz, J.; Bae, S.C.; Fortin, P.R.; et al. Soluble urokinase plasminogen activator receptor (suPAR) levels predict damage accrual in patients with recent-onset systemic lupus erythematosus. *J. Autoimmun.* **2020**, *106*, 102340. [CrossRef]
55. Dieker, J.; Berden, J.H.; Bakker, M.; Briand, J.P.; Muller, S.; Voll, R.; Sjöwall, C.; Herrmann, M.; Hilbrands, L.B.; van der Vlag, J. Autoantibodies against Modified Histone Peptides in SLE Patients Are Associated with Disease Activity and Lupus Nephritis. *PLoS ONE* **2016**, *11*, e0165373. [CrossRef]
56. Lu, J.; Marnell, L.L.; Marjon, K.D.; Mold, C.; Du Clos, T.W.; Sun, P.D. Structural recognition and functional activation of FcgammaR by innate pentraxins. *Nature* **2008**, *456*, 989–992. [CrossRef] [PubMed]
57. Ganrot, P.O.; Kindmark, C.O. C-reactive protein–a phagocytosis-promoting factor. *Scand J. Clin. Lab. Investig.* **1969**, *24*, 215–219. [CrossRef] [PubMed]
58. Mortensen, R.F.; Osmand, A.P.; Lint, T.F.; Gewurz, H. Interaction of C-reactive protein with lymphocytes and monocytes: Complement-dependent adherence and phagocytosis. *J. Immunol.* **1976**, *117*, 774–781.
59. Manderson, A.P.; Botto, M.; Walport, M.J. The role of complement in the development of systemic lupus erythematosus. *Annu. Rev. Immunol.* **2004**, *22*, 431–456. [CrossRef]
60. Truedsson, L.; Bengtsson, A.A.; Sturfelt, G. Complement deficiencies and systemic lupus erythematosus. *Autoimmunity* **2007**, *40*, 560–566. [CrossRef] [PubMed]
61. Kaplan, M.H.; Volanakis, J.E. Interaction of C-reactive protein complexes with the complement system. I. Consumption of human complement associated with the reaction of C-reactive protein with pneumococcal C-polysaccharide and with the choline phosphatides, lecithin and sphingomyelin. *J. Immunol.* **1974**, *112*, 2135–2147.
62. Siegel, J.; Rent, R.; Gewurz, H. Interactions of C-reactive protein with the complement system. I. Protamine-induced consumption of complement in acute phase sera. *J. Exp. Med.* **1974**, *140*, 631–647. [CrossRef]
63. Ji, S.R.; Wu, Y.; Potempa, L.A.; Liang, Y.H.; Zhao, J. Effect of modified C-reactive protein on complement activation: A possible complement regulatory role of modified or monomeric C-reactive protein in atherosclerotic lesions. *Arterioscler Thromb. Vasc. Biol.* **2006**, *26*, 935–941. [CrossRef] [PubMed]
64. Zeller, J.; Bogner, B.; Kiefer, J.; Braig, D.; Winninger, O.; Fricke, M.; Karasu, E.; Peter, K.; Huber-Lang, M.; Eisenhardt, S.U. CRP Enhances the Innate Killing Mechanisms Phagocytosis and ROS Formation in a Conformation and Complement-Dependent Manner. *Front. Immunol.* **2021**, *12*, 721887. [CrossRef]
65. Berman, S.; Gewurz, H.; Mold, C. Binding of C-reactive protein to nucleated cells leads to complement activation without cytolysis. *J. Immunol.* **1986**, *136*, 1354–1359.

66. Jarva, H.; Jokiranta, T.S.; Hellwage, J.; Zipfel, P.F.; Meri, S. Regulation of complement activation by C-reactive protein: Targeting the complement inhibitory activity of factor H by an interaction with short consensus repeat domains 7 and 8–11. *J. Immunol.* **1999**, *163*, 3957–3962.
67. Mold, C.; Gewurz, H.; Du Clos, T.W. Regulation of complement activation by C-reactive protein. *Immunopharmacology* **1999**, *42*, 23–30. [CrossRef]
68. Weiler, J.M.; Daha, M.R.; Austen, K.F.; Fearon, D.T. Control of the amplification convertase of complement by the plasma protein beta1H. *Proc. Natl. Acad. Sci USA* **1976**, *73*, 3268–3272. [CrossRef] [PubMed]
69. Whaley, K.; Ruddy, S. Modulation of the alternative complement pathways by beta 1 H globulin. *J. Exp. Med.* **1976**, *144*, 1147–1163. [CrossRef]
70. Harrison, R.A.; Lachmann, P.J. The physiological breakdown of the third component of human complement. *Mol. Immunol.* **1980**, *17*, 9–20. [CrossRef]
71. Pangburn, M.K.; Schreiber, R.D.; Muller-Eberhard, H.J. Human complement C3b inactivator: Isolation, characterization, and demonstration of an absolute requirement for the serum protein beta1H for cleavage of C3b and C4b in solution. *J. Exp. Med.* **1977**, *146*, 257–270. [CrossRef]
72. Mihlan, M.; Stippa, S.; Jozsi, M.; Zipfel, P.F. Monomeric CRP contributes to complement control in fluid phase and on cellular surfaces and increases phagocytosis by recruiting factor H. *Cell Death Differ.* **2009**, *16*, 1630–1640. [CrossRef]
73. Pang, Y.; Yang, X.W.; Song, Y.; Yu, F.; Zhao, M.H. Anti-C1q autoantibodies from active lupus nephritis patients could inhibit the clearance of apoptotic cells and complement classical pathway activation mediated by C1q in vitro. *Immunobiology* **2014**, *219*, 980–989. [CrossRef]
74. Trendelenburg, M.; Marfurt, J.; Gerber, I.; Tyndall, A.; Schifferli, J.A. Lack of occurrence of severe lupus nephritis among anti-C1q autoantibody-negative patients. *Arthritis. Rheum.* **1999**, *42*, 187–188. [CrossRef]
75. Janko, C.; Franz, S.; Munoz, L.E.; Siebig, S.; Winkler, S.; Schett, G.; Lauber, K.; Sheriff, A.; van der Vlag, J.; Herrmann, M. CRP/anti-CRP antibodies assembly on the surfaces of cell remnants switches their phagocytic clearance toward inflammation. *Front. Immunol.* **2011**, *2*, 70. [CrossRef] [PubMed]
76. Sjöwall, C.; Wetterö, J. Pathogenic implications for autoantibodies against C-reactive protein and other acute phase proteins. *Clin. Chim. Acta.* **2007**, *378*, 13–23. [CrossRef]
77. Gatto, M.; Radu, C.M.; Luisetto, R.; Ghirardello, A.; Bonsembiante, F.; Trez, D.; Valentino, S.; Bottazzi, B.; Simioni, P.; Cavicchioli, L.; et al. Immunization with Pentraxin3 prevents transition from subclinical to clinical lupus nephritis in lupus-prone mice: Insights from renal ultrastructural findings. *J. Autoimmun.* **2020**, *111*, 102443. [CrossRef]
78. Sjöwall, C.; Olin, A.I.; Skogh, T.; Wetterö, J.; Morgelin, M.; Nived, O.; Sturfelt, G.; Bengtsson, A.A. C-reactive protein, immunoglobulin G and complement co-localize in renal immune deposits of proliferative lupus nephritis. *Autoimmunity* **2013**, *46*, 205–214. [CrossRef]
79. Li, Q.Y.; Li, H.Y.; Fu, G.; Yu, F.; Wu, Y.; Zhao, M.H. Autoantibodies against C-Reactive Protein Influence Complement Activation and Clinical Course in Lupus Nephritis. *J. Am. Soc. Nephrol.* **2017**, *28*, 3044–3054. [CrossRef] [PubMed]
80. Tan, M.; Hao, J.B.; Chu, H.; Wang, F.M.; Song, D.; Zhu, L.; Yu, F.; Li, Y.Z.; Song, Y.; Zhao, M.H. Genetic variants in FH are associated with renal histopathologic subtypes of lupus nephritis: A large cohort study from China. *Lupus* **2017**, *26*, 1309–1317. [CrossRef]
81. Wang, F.M.; Song, D.; Pang, Y.; Song, Y.; Yu, F.; Zhao, M.H. The dysfunctions of complement factor H in lupus nephritis. *Lupus* **2016**, *25*, 1328–1340. [CrossRef] [PubMed]
82. Karpati, E.; Papp, A.; Schneider, A.E.; Hajnal, D.; Cserhalmi, M.; Csincsi, A.I.; Uzonyi, B.; Jozsi, M. Interaction of the Factor H Family Proteins FHR-1 and FHR-5 With DNA and Dead Cells: Implications for the Regulation of Complement Activation and Opsonization. *Front Immunol.* **2020**, *11*, 1297. [CrossRef] [PubMed]
83. Hebecker, M.; Okemefuna, A.I.; Perkins, S.J.; Mihlan, M.; Huber-Lang, M.; Jozsi, M. Molecular basis of C-reactive protein binding and modulation of complement activation by factor H-related protein 4. *Mol. Immunol.* **2010**, *47*, 1347–1355. [CrossRef] [PubMed]
84. Mihlan, M.; Hebecker, M.; Dahse, H.M.; Halbich, S.; Huber-Lang, M.; Dahse, R.; Zipfel, P.F.; Jozsi, M. Human complement factor H-related protein 4 binds and recruits native pentameric C-reactive protein to necrotic cells. *Mol. Immunol.* **2009**, *46*, 335–344. [CrossRef]
85. Mihlan, M.; Blom, A.M.; Kupreishvili, K.; Lauer, N.; Stelzner, K.; Bergström, F.; Niessen, H.W.; Zipfel, P.F. Monomeric C-reactive protein modulates classic complement activation on necrotic cells. *FASEB J.* **2011**, *25*, 4198–4210. [CrossRef] [PubMed]
86. Sjöberg, A.P.; Trouw, L.A.; McGrath, F.D.; Hack, C.E.; Blom, A.M. Regulation of complement activation by C-reactive protein: Targeting of the inhibitory activity of C4b-binding protein. *J. Immunol.* **2006**, *176*, 7612–7620. [CrossRef]
87. Sjöwall, C.; Wetterö, J.; Bengtsson, T.; Askendal, A.; Almroth, G.; Skogh, T.; Tengvall, P. Solid-phase classical complement activation by C-reactive protein (CRP) is inhibited by fluid-phase CRP-C1q interaction. *Biochem. Biophys. Res. Commun.* **2007**, *352*, 251–258. [CrossRef]
88. Roy, N.; Ohtani, K.; Matsuda, Y.; Mori, K.; Hwang, I.; Suzuki, Y.; Inoue, N.; Wakamiya, N. Collectin CL-P1 utilizes C-reactive protein for complement activation. *Biochim. Biophys Acta.* **2016**, *1860*, 1118–1128. [CrossRef]
89. Lu, J.; Mold, C.; Du Clos, T.W.; Sun, P.D. Pentraxins and Fc Receptor-Mediated Immune Responses. *Front Immunol.* **2018**, *9*, 2607. [CrossRef]

90. Bharadwaj, D.; Stein, M.P.; Volzer, M.; Mold, C.; Du Clos, T.W. The major receptor for C-reactive protein on leukocytes is fcgamma receptor II. *J. Exp. Med.* **1999**, *190*, 585–590. [CrossRef]
91. Manolov, D.E.; Rocker, C.; Hombach, V.; Nienhaus, G.U.; Torzewski, J. Ultrasensitive confocal fluorescence microscopy of C-reactive protein interacting with FcgammaRIIa. *Arterioscler. Thromb. Vasc. Biol.* **2004**, *24*, 2372–2377. [CrossRef] [PubMed]
92. Mold, C.; Du Clos, T.W. C-reactive protein increases cytokine responses to Streptococcus pneumoniae through interactions with Fc gamma receptors. *J. Immunol.* **2006**, *176*, 7598–7604. [CrossRef] [PubMed]
93. Båve, U.; Magnusson, M.; Eloranta, M.L.; Perers, A.; Alm, G.V.; Rönnblom, L. Fc gamma RIIa is expressed on natural IFN-alpha-producing cells (plasmacytoid dendritic cells) and is required for the IFN-alpha production induced by apoptotic cells combined with lupus IgG. *J. Immunol.* **2003**, *171*, 3296–3302. [CrossRef] [PubMed]
94. Mold, C.; Clos, T.W. C-reactive protein inhibits plasmacytoid dendritic cell interferon responses to autoantibody immune complexes. *Arthritis. Rheum.* **2013**, *65*, 1891–1901. [CrossRef]
95. Lu, J.; Marjon, K.D.; Marnell, L.L.; Wang, R.; Mold, C.; Du Clos, T.W.; Sun, P. Recognition and functional activation of the human IgA receptor (FcalphaRI) by C-reactive protein. *Proc. Natl. Acad. Sci. USA* **2011**, *108*, 4974–4979. [CrossRef]
96. Calabro, P.; Willerson, J.T.; Yeh, E.T. Inflammatory cytokines stimulated C-reactive protein production by human coronary artery smooth muscle cells. *Circulation* **2003**, *108*, 1930–1932. [CrossRef]
97. Gould, J.M.; Weiser, J.N. Expression of C-reactive protein in the human respiratory tract. *Infect. Immun.* **2001**, *69*, 1747–1754. [CrossRef]
98. Hernandez-Caldera, A.; Vernal, R.; Paredes, R.; Veloso-Matta, P.; Astorga, J.; Hernandez, M. Human periodontal ligament fibroblasts synthesize C-reactive protein and Th-related cytokines in response to interleukin (IL)-6 trans-signalling. *Int. Endod. J.* **2018**, *51*, 632–640. [CrossRef]
99. Jabs, W.J.; Logering, B.A.; Gerke, P.; Kreft, B.; Wolber, E.M.; Klinger, M.H.; Fricke, L.; Steinhoff, J. The kidney as a second site of human C-reactive protein formation in vivo. *Eur. J. Immunol.* **2003**, *33*, 152–161. [CrossRef] [PubMed]
100. Li, M.; Liu, J.; Han, C.; Wang, B.; Pang, X.; Mao, J. Angiotensin II induces the expression of c-reactive protein via MAPK-dependent signal pathway in U937 macrophages. *Cell Physiol. Biochem.* **2011**, *27*, 63–70. [CrossRef]
101. Zhang, D.; Jiang, S.L.; Rzewnicki, D.; Samols, D.; Kushner, I. The effect of interleukin-1 on C-reactive protein expression in Hep3B cells is exerted at the transcriptional level. *Biochem. J.* **1995**, *310*, 143–148. [CrossRef]
102. Zhang, D.; Sun, M.; Samols, D.; Kushner, I. STAT3 participates in transcriptional activation of the C-reactive protein gene by interleukin-6. *J. Biol. Chem.* **1996**, *271*, 9503–9509. [CrossRef]
103. Agrawal, A.; Cha-Molstad, H.; Samols, D.; Kushner, I. Transactivation of C-reactive protein by IL-6 requires synergistic interaction of CCAAT/enhancer binding protein beta (C/EBP beta) and Rel p50. *J. Immunol.* **2001**, *166*, 2378–2384. [CrossRef] [PubMed]
104. Enocsson, H.; Sjöwall, C.; Skogh, T.; Eloranta, M.L.; Rönnblom, L.; Wetterö, J. Interferon-alpha mediates suppression of C-reactive protein: Explanation for muted C-reactive protein response in lupus flares? *Arthritis. Rheum.* **2009**, *60*, 3755–3760. [CrossRef]
105. Gabay, C.; Genin, B.; Mentha, G.; Iynedjian, P.B.; Roux-Lombard, P.; Guerne, P.A. IL-1 receptor antagonist (IL-1Ra) does not inhibit the production of C-reactive protein or serum amyloid A protein by human primary hepatocytes. Differential regulation in normal and tumour cells. *Clin. Exp. Immunol.* **1995**, *100*, 306–313. [CrossRef] [PubMed]
106. Pepys, M.B.; Lanham, J.G.; De Beer, F.C. C-reactive protein in SLE. *Clin Rheum Dis* **1982**, *8*, 91–103. [CrossRef]
107. Rönnblom, L.; Eloranta, M.L. The interferon signature in autoimmune diseases. *Curr. Opin. Rheumatol.* **2013**, *25*, 248–253. [CrossRef] [PubMed]
108. Nakayama, T.; Sonoda, S.; Urano, T.; Yamada, T.; Okada, M. Monitoring both serum amyloid protein A and C-reactive protein as inflammatory markers in infectious diseases. *Clin. Chem.* **1993**, *39*, 293–297. [CrossRef]
109. Eloranta, M.L.; Rönnblom, L. Cause and consequences of the activated type I interferon system in SLE. *J. Mol. Med.* **2016**, *94*, 1103–1110. [CrossRef]
110. de Weerd, N.A.; Nguyen, T. The interferons and their receptors–distribution and regulation. *Immunol. Cell Biol.* **2012**, *90*, 483–491. [CrossRef] [PubMed]
111. Enocsson, H.; Sjöwall, C.; Kastbom, A.; Skogh, T.; Eloranta, M.L.; Rönnblom, L.; Wetterö, J. Association of serum C-reactive protein levels with lupus disease activity in the absence of measurable interferon-alpha and a C-reactive protein gene variant. *Arthritis. Rheumatol.* **2014**, *66*, 1568–1573. [CrossRef]
112. Hage, F.G.; Szalai, A.J. C-reactive protein gene polymorphisms, C-reactive protein blood levels, and cardiovascular disease risk. *J. Am. Coll. Cardiol.* **2007**, *50*, 1115–1122. [CrossRef] [PubMed]
113. Szalai, A.J.; Alarcon, G.S.; Calvo-Alen, J.; Toloza, S.M.; McCrory, M.A.; Edberg, J.C.; McGwin, G., Jr.; Bastian, H.M.; Fessler, B.J.; Vila, L.M.; et al. Systemic lupus erythematosus in a multiethnic US Cohort (LUMINA). XXX: Association between C-reactive protein (CRP) gene polymorphisms and vascular events. *Rheumatology* **2005**, *44*, 864–868. [CrossRef]
114. Szalai, A.J.; Wu, J.; Lange, E.M.; McCrory, M.A.; Langefeld, C.D.; Williams, A.; Zakharkin, S.O.; George, V.; Allison, D.B.; Cooper, G.S.; et al. Single-nucleotide polymorphisms in the C-reactive protein (CRP) gene promoter that affect transcription factor binding, alter transcriptional activity, and associate with differences in baseline serum CRP level. *J. Mol. Med.* **2005**, *83*, 440–447. [CrossRef] [PubMed]
115. Enocsson, H.; Gullstrand, B.; Eloranta, M.L.; Wetterö, J.; Leonard, D.; Rönnblom, L.; Bengtsson, A.A.; Sjöwall, C. C-Reactive Protein Levels in Systemic Lupus Erythematosus Are Modulated by the Interferon Gene Signature and CRP Gene Polymorphism rs1205. *Front. Immunol.* **2021**, *11*, 622326. [CrossRef]

116. Potempa, L.A.; Maldonado, B.A.; Laurent, P.; Zemel, E.S.; Gewurz, H. Antigenic, electrophoretic and binding alterations of human C-reactive protein modified selectively in the absence of calcium. *Mol. Immunol.* **1983**, *20*, 1165–1175. [CrossRef]
117. Verma, S.; Szmitko, P.E.; Yeh, E.T. C-reactive protein: Structure affects function. *Circulation* **2004**, *109*, 1914–1917. [CrossRef]
118. Ji, S.R.; Wu, Y.; Zhu, L.; Potempa, L.A.; Sheng, F.L.; Lu, W.; Zhao, J. Cell membranes and liposomes dissociate C-reactive protein (CRP) to form a new, biologically active structural intermediate: mCRP(m). *FASEB J.* **2007**, *21*, 284–294. [CrossRef]
119. Potempa, L.A.; Siegel, J.N.; Fiedel, B.A.; Potempa, R.T.; Gewurz, H. Expression, detection and assay of a neoantigen (Neo-CRP) associated with a free, human C-reactive protein subunit. *Mol. Immunol.* **1987**, *24*, 531–541. [CrossRef]
120. Schwedler, S.B.; Filep, J.G.; Galle, J.; Wanner, C.; Potempa, L.A. C-reactive protein: A family of proteins to regulate cardiovascular function. *Am. J. Kidney. Dis.* **2006**, *47*, 212–222. [CrossRef]
121. Skogh, T.; Stendahl, O. Complement-mediated delay in immune complex clearance from the blood owing to reduced deposition outside the reticuloendothelial system. *Immunology* **1983**, *49*, 53–59.
122. Motie, M.; Brockmeier, S.; Potempa, L.A. Binding of model soluble immune complexes to modified C-reactive protein. *J. Immunol.* **1996**, *156*, 4435–4441. [PubMed]
123. Eisenhardt, S.U.; Habersberger, J.; Murphy, A.; Chen, Y.C.; Woollard, K.J.; Bassler, N.; Qian, H.; von Zur Muhlen, C.; Hagemeyer, C.E.; Ahrens, I.; et al. Dissociation of pentameric to monomeric C-reactive protein on activated platelets localizes inflammation to atherosclerotic plaques. *Circ. Res.* **2009**, *105*, 128–137. [CrossRef] [PubMed]
124. Li, H.Y.; Liu, X.L.; Liu, Y.T.; Jia, Z.K.; Filep, J.G.; Potempa, L.A.; Ji, S.R.; Wu, Y. Matrix sieving-enforced retrograde transcytosis regulates tissue accumulation of C-reactive protein. *Cardiovasc Res.* **2019**, *115*, 440–452. [CrossRef] [PubMed]
125. Iso, H.; Cui, R.; Date, C.; Kikuchi, S.; Tamakoshi, A.; Group, J.S. C-reactive protein levels and risk of mortality from cardiovascular disease in Japanese: The JACC Study. *Atherosclerosis* **2009**, *207*, 291–297. [CrossRef]
126. Ji, S.R.; Wu, Y.; Potempa, L.A.; Qiu, Q.; Zhao, J. Interactions of C-reactive protein with low-density lipoproteins: Implications for an active role of modified C-reactive protein in atherosclerosis. *Int. J. Biochem. Cell Biol.* **2006**, *38*, 648–661. [CrossRef]
127. Jiang, S.; Bao, Y.; Hou, X.; Fang, Q.; Wang, C.; Pan, J.; Zuo, Y.; Zhong, W.; Xiang, K.; Jia, W. Serum C-reactive protein and risk of cardiovascular events in middle-aged and older chinese population. *Am. J. Cardiol.* **2009**, *103*, 1727–1731. [CrossRef]
128. Molins, B.; Pena, E.; Vilahur, G.; Mendieta, C.; Slevin, M.; Badimon, L. C-reactive protein isoforms differ in their effects on thrombus growth. *Arterioscler. Thromb Vasc. Biol.* **2008**, *28*, 2239–2246. [CrossRef]
129. Ridker, P.M.; Paynter, N.P.; Rifai, N.; Gaziano, J.M.; Cook, N.R. C-reactive protein and parental history improve global cardiovascular risk prediction: The Reynolds Risk Score for men. *Circulation* **2008**, *118*, 2243–2251. [CrossRef] [PubMed]
130. Ridker, P.M.; Danielson, E.; Fonseca, F.A.; Genest, J.; Gotto, A.M., Jr.; Kastelein, J.J.; Koenig, W.; Libby, P.; Lorenzatti, A.J.; MacFadyen, J.G.; et al. Rosuvastatin to prevent vascular events in men and women with elevated C-reactive protein. *N Engl. J. Med.* **2008**, *359*, 2195–2207. [CrossRef] [PubMed]
131. Habersberger, J.; Strang, F.; Scheichl, A.; Htun, N.; Bassler, N.; Merivirta, R.M.; Diehl, P.; Krippner, G.; Meikle, P.; Eisenhardt, S.U.; et al. Circulating microparticles generate and transport monomeric C-reactive protein in patients with myocardial infarction. *Cardiovasc Res.* **2012**, *96*, 64–72. [CrossRef]
132. Strang, F.; Scheichl, A.; Chen, Y.C.; Wang, X.; Htun, N.M.; Bassler, N.; Eisenhardt, S.U.; Habersberger, J.; Peter, K. Amyloid plaques dissociate pentameric to monomeric C-reactive protein: A novel pathomechanism driving cortical inflammation in Alzheimer's disease? *Brain Pathol.* **2012**, *22*, 337–346. [CrossRef]
133. Eisenhardt, S.U.; Thiele, J.R.; Bannasch, H.; Stark, G.B.; Peter, K. C-reactive protein: How conformational changes influence inflammatory properties. *Cell Cycle.* **2009**, *8*, 3885–3892. [CrossRef] [PubMed]
134. Ji, S.R.; Ma, L.; Bai, C.J.; Shi, J.M.; Li, H.Y.; Potempa, L.A.; Filep, J.G.; Zhao, J.; Wu, Y. Monomeric C-reactive protein activates endothelial cells via interaction with lipid raft microdomains. *FASEB J.* **2009**, *23*, 1806–1816. [CrossRef] [PubMed]
135. Khreiss, T.; Jozsef, L.; Hossain, S.; Chan, J.S.; Potempa, L.A.; Filep, J.G. Loss of pentameric symmetry of C-reactive protein is associated with delayed apoptosis of human neutrophils. *J. Biol. Chem.* **2002**, *277*, 40775–40781. [CrossRef] [PubMed]
136. Khreiss, T.; Jozsef, L.; Potempa, L.A.; Filep, J.G. Conformational rearrangement in C-reactive protein is required for proinflammatory actions on human endothelial cells. *Circulation* **2004**, *109*, 2016–2022. [CrossRef] [PubMed]
137. Khreiss, T.; Jozsef, L.; Potempa, L.A.; Filep, J.G. Opposing effects of C-reactive protein isoforms on shear-induced neutrophil-platelet adhesion and neutrophil aggregation in whole blood. *Circulation* **2004**, *110*, 2713–2720. [CrossRef]
138. Khreiss, T.; Jozsef, L.; Potempa, L.A.; Filep, J.G. Loss of pentameric symmetry in C-reactive protein induces interleukin-8 secretion through peroxynitrite signaling in human neutrophils. *Circ. Res.* **2005**, *97*, 690–697. [CrossRef] [PubMed]
139. Lauer, N.; Mihlan, M.; Hartmann, A.; Schlotzer-Schrehardt, U.; Keilhauer, C.; Scholl, H.P.; Charbel Issa, P.; Holz, F.; Weber, B.H.; Skerka, C.; et al. Complement regulation at necrotic cell lesions is impaired by the age-related macular degeneration-associated factor-H His402 risk variant. *J. Immunol.* **2011**, *187*, 4374–4383. [CrossRef]
140. Molins, B.; Pena, E.; de la Torre, R.; Badimon, L. Monomeric C-reactive protein is prothrombotic and dissociates from circulating pentameric C-reactive protein on adhered activated platelets under flow. *Cardiovasc. Res.* **2011**, *92*, 328–337. [CrossRef] [PubMed]
141. Wang, M.Y.; Ji, S.R.; Bai, C.J.; El Kebir, D.; Li, H.Y.; Shi, J.M.; Zhu, W.; Costantino, S.; Zhou, H.H.; Potempa, L.A.; et al. A redox switch in C-reactive protein modulates activation of endothelial cells. *FASEB J.* **2011**, *25*, 3186–3196. [CrossRef] [PubMed]
142. Zouki, C.; Haas, B.; Chan, J.S.; Potempa, L.A.; Filep, J.G. Loss of pentameric symmetry of C-reactive protein is associated with promotion of neutrophil-endothelial cell adhesion. *J. Immunol.* **2001**, *167*, 5355–5361. [CrossRef] [PubMed]

143. Boncler, M.; Kehrel, B.; Szewczyk, R.; Stec-Martyna, E.; Bednarek, R.; Brodde, M.; Watala, C. Oxidation of C-reactive protein by hypochlorous acid leads to the formation of potent platelet activator. *Int. J. Biol. Macromol.* **2018**, *107*, 2701–2714. [CrossRef]
144. Schwedler, S.B.; Guderian, F.; Dammrich, J.; Potempa, L.A.; Wanner, C. Tubular staining of modified C-reactive protein in diabetic chronic kidney disease. *Nephrol. Dial. Transplant* **2003**, *18*, 2300–2307. [CrossRef] [PubMed]
145. Slevin, M.; Matou-Nasri, S.; Turu, M.; Luque, A.; Rovira, N.; Badimon, L.; Boluda, S.; Potempa, L.; Sanfeliu, C.; de Vera, N.; et al. Modified C-reactive protein is expressed by stroke neovessels and is a potent activator of angiogenesis in vitro. *Brain Pathol.* **2010**, *20*, 151–165. [CrossRef] [PubMed]
146. Robey, F.A.; Jones, K.D.; Steinberg, A.D. C-reactive protein mediates the solubilization of nuclear DNA by complement in vitro. *J. Exp. Med.* **1985**, *161*, 1344–1356. [CrossRef]
147. Bell, S.A.; Du Clos, T.W.; Khursigara, G.; Picazo, J.J.; Rubin, R.L. Autoantibodies to cryptic epitopes of C-reactive protein and other acute phase proteins in the toxic oil syndrome. *J. Autoimmun.* **1995**, *8*, 293–303. [CrossRef]
148. Bell, S.A.; Faust, H.; Schmid, A.; Meurer, M. Autoantibodies to C-reactive protein (CRP) and other acute-phase proteins in systemic autoimmune diseases. *Clin. Exp. Immunol.* **1998**, *113*, 327–332. [CrossRef]
149. Sjöwall, C.; Eriksson, P.; Almer, S.; Skogh, T. Autoantibodies to C-reactive protein is a common finding in SLE, but not in primary Sjogren's syndrome, rheumatoid arthritis or inflammatory bowel disease. *J. Autoimmun.* **2002**, *19*, 155–160. [CrossRef]
150. Sjöwall, C.; Bengtsson, A.A.; Sturfelt, G.; Skogh, T. Serum levels of autoantibodies against monomeric C-reactive protein are correlated with disease activity in systemic lupus erythematosus. *Arthritis. Res. Ther.* **2004**, *6*, R87–R94. [CrossRef]
151. Rosenau, B.J.; Schur, P.H. Antibodies to C reactive protein. *Ann. Rheum. Dis.* **2006**, *65*, 674–676. [CrossRef]
152. Sjöwall, C.; Cardell, K.; Boström, E.A.; Bokarewa, M.I.; Enocsson, H.; Ekstedt, M.; Lindvall, L.; Fryden, A.; Almer, S. High prevalence of autoantibodies to C-reactive protein in patients with chronic hepatitis C infection: Association with liver fibrosis and portal inflammation. *Hum. Immunol.* **2012**, *73*, 382–388. [CrossRef] [PubMed]
153. Jakuszko, K.; Krajewska, M.; Halon, A.; Koscielska-Kasprzak, K.; Myszka, M.; Zabinska, M.; Augustyniak-Bartosik, H.; Rukasz, D.; Weyde, W.; Klinger, M. Pathogenic role of antibodies against monomeric C-reactive protein in tubulointerstitial nephritis and uveitis syndrome. *Intern. Med. J.* **2014**, *44*, 809–812. [CrossRef]
154. Figueredo, M.A.; Rodriguez, A.; Ruiz-Yague, M.; Romero, M.; Fernandez-Cruz, A.; Gomez-de la Concha, E.; Patino, R. Autoantibodies against C-reactive protein: Clinical associations in systemic lupus erythematosus and primary antiphospholipid syndrome. *J. Rheumatol.* **2006**, *33*, 1980–1986. [PubMed]
155. Pesickova, S.S.; Rysava, R.; Lenicek, M.; Vitek, L.; Potlukova, E.; Hruskova, Z.; Jancova, E.; Honsova, E.; Zavada, J.; Trendelenburg, M.; et al. Prognostic value of anti-CRP antibodies in lupus nephritis in long-term follow-up. *Arthritis Res. Ther.* **2015**, *17*, 371. [CrossRef]
156. Mathsson, L.; Ahlin, E.; Sjöwall, C.; Skogh, T.; Rönnelid, J. Cytokine induction by circulating immune complexes and signs of in-vivo complement activation in systemic lupus erythematosus are associated with the occurrence of anti-Sjogren's syndrome A antibodies. *Clin. Exp. Immunol.* **2007**, *147*, 513–520. [CrossRef]
157. O'Neill, S.G.; Giles, I.; Lambrianides, A.; Manson, J.; D'Cruz, D.; Schrieber, L.; March, L.M.; Latchman, D.S.; Isenberg, D.A.; Rahman, A. Antibodies to apolipoprotein A-I, high-density lipoprotein, and C-reactive protein are associated with disease activity in patients with systemic lupus erythematosus. *Arthritis Rheum.* **2010**, *62*, 845–854. [CrossRef] [PubMed]
158. Wener, M.H.; Uwatoko, S.; Mannik, M. Antibodies to the collagen-like region of C1q in sera of patients with autoimmune rheumatic diseases. *Arthritis Rheum.* **1989**, *32*, 544–551. [CrossRef] [PubMed]

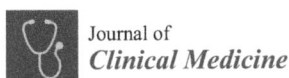

Article

CRP Serum Levels Are Associated with High Cardiometabolic Risk and Clinical Disease Activity in Systemic Lupus Erythematosus Patients

Karen Pesqueda-Cendejas [1,2], Isela Parra-Rojas [1,3], Paulina E. Mora-García [1,2], Margarita Montoya-Buelna [1,4], Adolfo I. Ruiz-Ballesteros [1,2], Mónica R. Meza-Meza [1,2], Bertha Campos-López [1,2], Melissa Rivera-Escoto [1,2], Barbara Vizmanos-Lamotte [1,2], Sergio Cerpa-Cruz [5] and Ulises de la Cruz-Mosso [1,2,*]

[1] Proyecto Inmunonutrición y Genómica Nutricional en las Enfermedades Autoinmunes, Centro Universitario de Ciencias de la Salud, Universidad de Guadalajara, Guadalajara 44340, Mexico; karen.pesqueda20@gmail.com (K.P.-C.); iprojas@yahoo.com (I.P.-R.); moragarciapaulinaesmeralda@gmail.com (P.E.M.-G.); margaritamontoyabuelna@gmail.com (M.M.-B.); adolfo.ruba@gmail.com (A.I.R.-B.); monimez28@hotmail.com (M.R.M.-M.); bertha.campos@live.com (B.C.-L.); melissa.rivera.e@hotmail.com (M.R.-E.); bvizmanos@yahoo.com.mx (B.V.-L.)
[2] Instituto de Nutrigenética y Nutrigenómica Traslacional, Centro Universitario de Ciencias de la Salud, Universidad de Guadalajara, Guadalajara 44340, Mexico
[3] Laboratorio de Investigación en Obesidad y Diabetes, Facultad de Ciencias Químico-Biológicas, Universidad Autónoma de Guerrero, Chilpancingo de los Bravo 39087, Mexico
[4] Laboratorio de Inmunología, Departamento de Fisiología, Centro Universitario de Ciencias de la Salud, Universidad de Guadalajara, Guadalajara 44340, Mexico
[5] Departamento de Reumatología, O.P.D. Hospital Civil de Guadalajara Fray Antonio Alcalde, Guadalajara 44280, Mexico; sacer04@prodigy.net.mx
* Correspondence: ulises_cdm@hotmail.com or ulises.mosso@academicos.udg.mx; Tel.: +52-1-331-744-15-75

Abstract: Systemic lupus erythematosus (SLE) patients have a higher frequency of cardiovascular risk factors such as high C-reactive protein (CRP) levels than the general population. CRP is considered a cardiovascular disease marker that could be related to SLE clinical disease activity. This study aimed to assess the association between CRP with cardiometabolic risk and clinical disease activity in SLE patients. A comparative cross-sectional study was conducted in 176 female SLE patients and 175 control subjects (CS) with median ages of 38 and 33 years, respectively; SLE patients were classified by the 1997 SLE-ACR criteria, and the clinical disease activity by the Mexican-SLEDAI (Mex-SLEDAI). CRP and lipid profile (triglycerides, cholesterol, HDL-C, and LDL-C) were quantified by turbidimetry and colorimetric-enzymatic assays, respectively. SLE patients had higher CRP levels than CS (SLE: 5 mg/L vs. CS = 1.1 mg/L; $p < 0.001$). In SLE patients, CRP levels ≥ 3 mg/L were associated with a higher risk of cardiometabolic risk status assessed by LAP index (OR = 3.01; IC: 1.04–8.7; $p = 0.04$), triglycerides/HDL-C index (OR = 5.2; IC: 2.1–12.8; $p < 0.001$), Kannel index (OR = 3.1; IC: 1.1–8.1; $p = 0.03$), Castelli index (OR = 6.6; IC: 2.5–17.8; $p < 0.001$), and high clinical disease activity (OR = 2.5: IC: 1.03–6.2; $p = 0.04$; and β coefficient = 5.8; IC: 2.5–9.4; R^2 = 0.15; $p = 0.001$). In conclusion, high CRP levels were associated with high cardiometabolic risk and clinical disease activity in SLE patients.

Keywords: C-reactive protein; cardiovascular risk; systemic lupus erythematosus; clinical activity; lipid profile; body composition

---

1. Introduction

Systemic lupus erythematosus (SLE) is a prototypical chronic autoimmune inflammatory disease characterized by the production of autoantibodies against self-antigens such as deoxyribonucleic acid (DNA), proteins, and nucleosomes [1], where genetic, environmental, and hormonal factors are involved. However, the exact mechanism of its

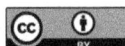

pathogenesis remains unknown [2]. The breakdown of self-tolerance and the altered innate responses against self-antigen induce antibody production, leading to the deposition of immune complexes in tissues and complement activation. These aberrant mechanisms are considered to be responsible for the clinical manifestations in SLE patients [2].

In SLE, mortality presents a bimodal pattern, with an initial peak due to clinical disease activity and a late peak attributable to the development of cardiovascular disorders [3]. Cardiovascular disease (CVD) is one of the major causes of morbidity and mortality in SLE; it is related to traditional CVD risk factors such as dyslipidemia, obesity, and smoking. Additionally, non-traditional risk factors derived from the SLE pathophysiology, such as the glucocorticoid treatment, and inflammatory mediators such as type 1 interferons (IFN), tumor necrosis factor-alpha (TNF-α), and C-reactive protein (CRP) are involved in CVD development [4–6].

CRP, a liver-derived acute-phase protein produced by hepatocytes mainly in response to the inflammatory cytokine interleukin 6 (IL-6), is considered a sensitive biomarker of bacterial infections, cardiovascular events, and inflammatory conditions [7]. The physiological functions of CRP are to increase phagocytosis and activate the classical pathway of the complement, which supports complex immune clearance. In healthy individuals, CRP circulates at low concentrations; its levels increase considerably in response to infection, tissue injury, and inflammation [8]. CRP has been suggested as a powerful predictor of CVD independent of other factors in the general population. It has a relevant role in atherosclerotic plaque formation, maturation, destabilization, and rupture; therefore, CRP is described as a predictor for arterial thrombotic events and tissue damage [7,8]. Recently, CRP apheresis has been suggested as an alternative translational therapy to reduce CRP levels and tissue damage, using a phosphocholine-derivative matrix as a ligand for CRP, which could be useful to selectively deplete CRP from blood plasma in patients recovering from acute myocardial infarction [9], and other inflammatory conditions such as SLE.

Concerning the pathogenic role of CRP in autoimmune diseases, it has been reported that SLE patients could have higher CRP serum levels compared to healthy controls [10], and the CRP serum levels correlate with traditional cardiovascular risk factors such as dyslipidemia, obesity, and glucose disturbances, which could be associated with a negative impact on robust outcomes such as damage, disease activity, and survival in SLE [11].

However, CRP's role in active SLE is still complex and controversial, some studies have reported that CRP levels are normal or modestly elevated in active SLE, and that there is no relationship between CRP levels and clinical disease activity [12,13]. Nevertheless, it is widely described that in active SLE patients there is an increase in inflammatory cytokines such as IL-6, which could directly drive the CRP serum levels, suggesting a potential relationship between the increase in IL-6 in the active SLE and higher CRP serum levels [7]. Previous studies have described that CRP serum levels correlate with clinical disease activity when evaluated by the SLEDAI-2K index, where it is proposed that CRP levels could reflect the clinical disease activity in SLE [11]. Notably, SLE patients have high cardiometabolic risk, which has been related to a high clinical disease activity [14]. Therefore, based on these previous findings, our study aimed to assess the association of CRP levels with cardiometabolic risk and clinical disease activity in SLE patients.

2. Materials and Methods

2.1. Subjects

We performed a comparative cross-sectional study on 176 female SLE patients from an unrelated Mexican Mestizo population, classified according to the 1997 American College of Rheumatology (ACR) criteria for SLE [15], recruited in 2017–2020 from the Rheumatology Department of the Hospital Civil Fray Antonio Alcalde, Guadalajara, Jalisco, Mexico.

The Mexican-Systemic Lupus Erythematosus-Disease Activity Index (Mex-SLEDAI) was used to evaluate clinical disease activity [16]. The SLE participants were without a previous diagnosis of CVD, no recent infections, trauma, surgery, pregnancy, or other autoimmune systemic conditions not related to the SLE.

The control group was 175 women recruited from the same geographical area. These control subjects (CS) did not have any recent infections, trauma, surgery, pregnancy, or autoimmune conditions; also, they did not refer family history of autoimmune diseases.

2.2. Ethical Considerations

This study was approved by the Research Ethical Committee of the University of Guadalajara (CI-05018 CUCS-UdeG), based on the international ethical guidelines. All the participants gave written informed consent for their participation.

2.3. Anthropometric Evaluation and Their Definitions

The anthropometric evaluation involved measurements of weight, fat mass, and muscle mass, which were determined in the morning through the bioimpedance analysis prediction method (TANITA® Ironman™ body composition Monitor BC-549, Arlington Heights, IL, USA), and height was measured to the nearest 0.1 cm using a stadiometer (Seca, Hamburg, Germany). Waist and hip circumferences were measured twice using a flexible metal tape with an accuracy of ±0.1 cm (Lufkin® executive thinline W606ME, Missouri City, TX, USA), with the subject standing with feet together and arms crossed. Waist circumference was measured at the midpoint between the costal margin and iliac crest in the mid-axillary line in standing position at the end of a gentle expiration, and a hip circumference measurement was taken around the widest portion of the buttocks [17].

From these measurements, body mass index (BMI) was calculated (BMI = weight, kg/height^2, m^2) according to the NOM-043-SSA2-2012-MEX based on World Health Organization (WHO) criteria [18]. The waist to hip ratio (WHR) was calculated (WHR = waist circumference, cm /hip circumference, cm) and classified to assess the distribution of abdominal fat in gynecoid (<0.85) or android ($\geq$0.85); waist circumference was classified as high risk ($\geq$80 cm) or low risk (<80 cm) for metabolic complications; the Waist to height ratio (WHtR) was calculated (WHtR = waist, cm/height, cm) and a score $\geq$ 0.5 was classified as a risk for metabolic abnormalities, according to the WHO cutoff values [18–20].

2.4. Hs-CRP Quantification

The quantification of CRP was determined using a high-sensitivity turbidimetric latex immunoassay with the high sensitivity CRP (hs-CRP) kit (COD 31927, BioSystems®, Barcelona, Spain); the detection limit of the assay was 0.06 mg/L, and the measurement interval was 0.06–15 mg/L.

2.5. Biochemical Measurements

Blood serum was taken from the participants after an overnight fast of 12 h; glucose and lipid profiles (triglycerides, total cholesterol, HDL-C, and LDL-C) were determined using a piece of semi-automated equipment (Mindray-BS-240 Clinical Chemistry Analyzer, Shenzhen, China) and colorimetric enzymatic assays (BioSystems® kits, Barcelona, Spain).

2.6. Biochemical and Cardiometabolic Criteria Definitions

To evaluate the CVD risk, we applied cut-points for CRP levels at low risk (<1.0 mg/L), average risk ($\geq$1.0 to <3.0 mg/L), and high risk ($\geq$3.0 mg/L) based on the criteria of the Centers for Disease Control and Prevention and the American Heart Association [21]. Cardiometabolic indexes were calculated and interpreted according to formulas described in detail in a previous study by Campos-López et al. [14]: (a) Castelli index classified as low (<4.5), moderate ($\geq$4.5 to <7.0) and high ($\geq$7.0) CVD risk; (b) Kannel index classified as low (<3) and high ($\geq$3) CVD risk; (c) TG/HDL-C ratio classified as elevated a score $\geq$3 [22]; (d) cardiometabolic index (CMI score) [20] classified by tertiles (T): T1st (minimum value to <0.6069) of low CVD risk, T2nd ($\geq$0.6069 to <1.188) and T3rd ($\geq$1.188 to maximum value), these last two considered as medium and high CVD risk, respectively; (e) lipid accumulation products (LAP score) [23] were classified as: (T): T1st (minimum value to

<10.74) of low CVD risk, T2nd ($\geq$10.74 to <31.06) and T3rd ($\geq$31.06 to maximum value), these last two were considered as medium and high CVD risk, respectively.

2.7. Statistical Analysis

The statistical analyses were performed with the software STATA v 9.2 (College Station, TX, USA) and GraphPad Prism v 5.0 (San Diego, CA, USA). The statistical power was evaluated according to the calculation of sample size, performed with an estimated error margin of 2% with a confidence degree of 95%, and expected prevalence of 60% for dyslipidemia after three years of disease evolution time in SLE patients reported in previous studies [7,8]. The normal variable distribution was assessed by the Shapiro–Wilk test. For descriptive analysis, categorical variables are expressed as frequencies; continuous variables with nonparametric variables are expressed as medians and percentiles 5th–95th.

For inferential analysis, the Fisher χ^2 test was used to compare proportions. Mann–Whitney U test was used for nonparametric quantitative determinations of two groups, and for nonparametric quantitative determinations of three groups, Kruskal–Wallis test was applied. The discriminative capacity of CRP to differentiate between SLE patients vs. CS, and active vs. inactive SLE patients was calculated using a receiver operator characteristic (ROC) curve, and the area under the curve (AUC) from the receiver operating characteristic was calculated. To determine the correlations between CRP with cardiometabolic variables and clinical disease activity, we used Spearman correlation tests. The associations of CRP with cardiometabolic indexes and the clinical disease activity were determined by logistic regression models to estimate odds ratios, and by linear regression models to estimate β coefficients, using adjusted models. The differences were considered significant at a p value < 0.05.

3. Results

3.1. General Characteristics in SLE Patients and CS

A total of 176 female SLE patients with a median age of 38 years were evaluated. They presented a median of clinical disease activity of 0 (remission), 44% were active patients, and 56% were in remission; 33% of the patients had renal activity, and the median of disease duration was of 7 years. As a reference control group representative of the same population, a total of 175 CS women with a median age of 33 years were evaluated. SLE patients had higher weights (SLE = 67 vs. CS = 61.2 kg; $p < 0.001$) than CS and presented a circumference waist > 80 cm (SLE = 84 vs. CS = 76.7 cm; $p < 0.001$) classified as cardiovascular risk; additionally, SLE patients had a BMI > 25 kg/m^2 classified as overweight (SLE = 26.9 vs. 23.6 kg/m^2; $p < 0.001$), while CS had an adequate weight according to BMI. SLE patients, in addition, had higher WHR scores (SLE = 0.52 vs. CS = 0.47; $p < 0.001$) than CS. Regarding biochemical variables, SLE patients had higher levels of triglycerides (SLE = 117.2 vs. CS = 76 mg/dL); $p < 0.001$, and lower levels of HDL-C (SLE = 33.7 vs. CS = 50.9 mg/dL; $p < 0.001$), regarding the cardiometabolic indexes. SLE patients presented a higher score with regard to the Castelli atherogenic index (SLE = 4.8 vs. CS = 3.3; $p < 0.001$), Kannel index (SLE = 2.4 vs. CS = 1.8; $p < 0.001$), triglycerides/HDL-C ratio (SLE = 3.6 vs. CS = 1.4; $p < 0.001$), CMI score (SLE = 1.19 vs. CS = 0.7; $p < 0.001$), and LAP score (SLE = 29 vs. CS = 15; $p < 0.001$) than CS (Table 1). Concerning the SLE treatment, 52.5% of the patients received prednisone treatment with a median dose of 10 mg/day, 46% used chloroquine (CQ) with a median dose of 150 mg/day, and 30.5% hydroxychloroquine (HCQ) with a median dose of 200 mg/day; additionally, 32% were in treatment with antihypertensives (Table 1).

Table 1. General characteristics in SLE patients and CS.

Variable	SLE (n = 176)	CS (n = 175)	p Value
SLE clinical features			
Mex-SLEDAI (score) [a]	0 (0–8)	-	-
Mex-SLEDAI classification % (n)			
Clinical disease activity (≥2) [b]	44 (69/167)	-	-
Clinical remission (<2) [b]	56 (86/167)	-	-
Renal activity % (n)	33 (32/97)	-	-
Disease duration (years) [a]	7 (0.6–21)	-	-
Body composition			
Weight (kg) [a]	67 (49.6–96.9)	61.2 (46.6–86.5)	**<0.001**
Waist (cm) [a]	84 (67.2–104.2)	76.7 (61.5–105)	**<0.001**
BMI (kg/m^2) [a]	26.9 (19.5–37.5)	23.6 (18.6–34)	**<0.001**
WHR (score) [a]	0.83 (0.73–0.93)	0.77 (0.68–0.93)	**<0.001**
WHtR (score) [a]	0.52 (0.41–0.65)	0.47 (0.38–0.65)	**<0.001**
Muscle mass (kg) [a]	40.7 (35.9–50.5)	39.8 (35.4–45.8)	**0.01**
Fat mass (%) [c]	33.4 ± 8.48	32.1 ± 9	0.87
Biochemical data			
Glucose (mg/dL) [a]	87.2 (71.0–133)	87.8 (75.1–118)	0.74
Triglycerides (mg/dL) [a]	117.2 (49–242)	76 (38–198)	**<0.001**
Total cholesterol (mg/dL) [a]	168.8 (121–245)	169 (121–245)	0.40
HDL-C (mg/dL) [a]	33.7 (14–64)	50.9 (32–77)	**<0.001**
LDL-C (mg/dL) [a]	77.5 (46–142)	95 (59–158)	**<0.001**
Cardiometabolic indexes			
Castelli atherogenic index (TC/HDL-C) [a]	4.8 (2.5–13.9)	3.2 (2.17–13.8)	**<0.001**
Kannel index (LDL-C/HDL-C) [a]	2.4 (1.1–5.6)	1.84 (1–3.5)	**<0.001**
Triglycerides/HDL-C ratio (score) [a]	3.6 (1–15)	1.4 (0.6–5.1)	**<0.001**
CMI (score) [a]	1.19 (0.44–3.39)	0.7 (0.26–4.8)	**<0.001**
LAP (score) [a]	29 (6.2–76)	15 (2.3–89)	**<0.001**
Treatment			
Prednisone % (n) [b]	52.5 (93/177)	-	-
Prednisone dose (mg/day) [a]	10 (5 50)	-	-
Chloroquine % (n) [b]	46 (81/177)	-	-
Chloroquine dose (mg/day) [a]	150 (100–200)	-	-
Hydroxychloroquine % (n) [b]	30.5 (54/177)	-	-
Hydroxychloroquine dose (mg/day) [a]	200 (150–200)	-	-
Antihypertensives % (n) [b]	32 (19/60)	-	-

[a] Data shown as median (percentile: p5th–p95th), p value: U Mann–Whitney test. [b] Data shown as percentages (n). [c] Data shown as mean and standard deviation, p value: Student's t-test. The bold numbers indicate variables with significant differences. **SLE**: systemic lupus erythematosus patients; **CS**: control subjects; **BMI**: body mass index; **WHR**: waist to hip ratio; **WHtR**: waist to height ratio (cm/cm); **HDL-C**: high-density lipoprotein cholesterol; **LDL-C**: low-density lipoprotein cholesterol; **TC**: total cholesterol; **CMI**: cardiometabolic index; CMI = (triglycerides/HDL-C); **LAP**: lipid accumulation products; LAP = (waist in cm − 58)*(triglycerides mmol/L).

3.2. CRP Levels and Cardiovascular Risk in Active and Inactive SLE

Concerning the CRP levels, SLE patients showed higher levels than the CS group (SLE = 5 vs. CS = 1.1 mg/L; $p \leq 0.001$) (Figure 1a); then, we determined the CRP capacity to discriminate between SLE patients and CS using ROC curves. Based on these results, the CRP levels have a high capacity of discrimination with an AUC of 0.73 (CI: 0.68–0.79; $p < 0.001$) (Figure 1b). When comparing CRP levels between active SLE and inactive SLE, we observed that active SLE patients have higher CRP levels than inactive SLE (active SLE = 6.2 vs. inactive SLE = 3.6 mg/L; $p < 0.001$) (Figure 1c). The CRP levels showed a moderate capacity to discriminate between active and inactive SLE with an AUC of 0.67 (CI: 0.58–0.75; $p < 0.001$) (Figure 1d).

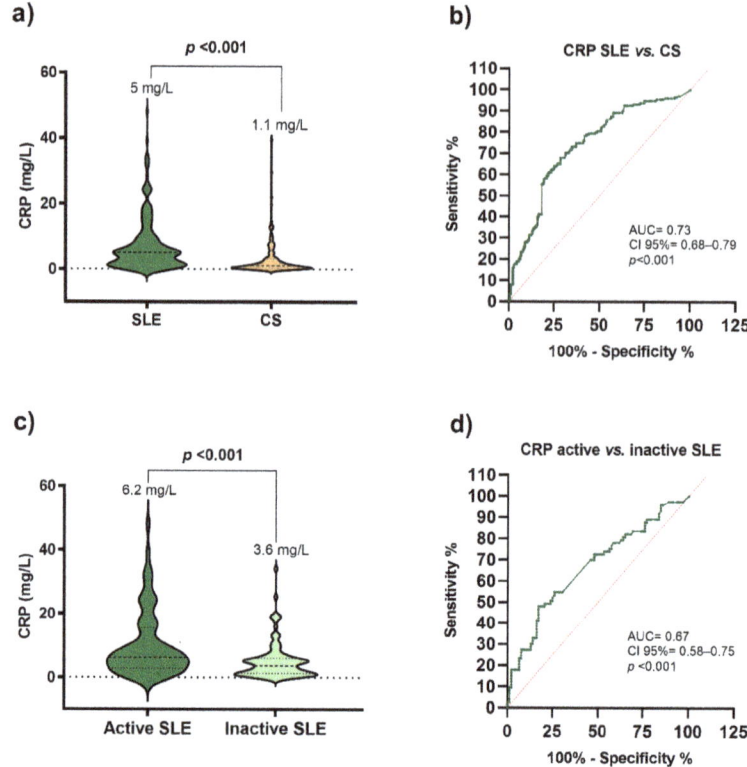

Figure 1. Serum CRP levels were stratified by study groups. (**a**) Serum CRP levels in SLE patients and CS. Data presented as median; p value U Mann–Whitney test. SLE: systemic lupus erythematosus patients; CS: control subjects; CRP: C-reactive protein. (**b**) Discriminatory receiver operating characteristic (ROC) curve between SLE patients vs. CS. AUC = area under the curve. 95% CI = 95% confidence interval. (**c**) Serum CRP levels stratified by clinical disease activity in SLE patients. Clinical inactivity: Mex-SLEDAI < 2; Clinical activity: Mex-SLEDAI ≥ 2. Data provided in median; p value U Mann–Whitney test. (**d**) Discriminatory receiver operating characteristic (ROC) curve between inactive vs. active SLE patients.

3.3. Biochemical and Cardiometabolic Status and CRP in SLE Patients and CS

To compare the biochemical and cardiometabolic statuses according to the CVD risk by the criteria from the center for disease control and prevention and the American Heart Association to CRP serum levels, both SLE patients and CS were stratified according to CRP levels as low CVD risk (<1 mg/dL), average CVD risk (≥1 to <3 mg/dL) and high CVD risk (≥3 mg/L). SLE patients with high CVD risk showed higher triglycerides levels ($p < 0.001$) and lower HDL-C levels ($p < 0.001$) than patients with low and average CVD risk; additionally, it was observed that SLE patients with levels of CRP ≥ 3 mg/L (high CVD risk) presented higher scores with regard to the Castelli index (6.5; $p < 0.001$), Kannel index (2.5; $p < 0.001$), triglycerides/HDL-C ratio (4.4; $p < 0.001$), CMI (1.4; $p = 0.03$) and LAP score (41.7; $p = 0.02$) (Table 2). SLE patients with levels of CRP ≥ 3 mg/L also presented a higher frequency for high CVD risk according to the Castelli index (48%; $p < 0.001$), Kannel index (40.4%; $p = 0.001$) and triglycerides/HDL-C ratio (71%; $p < 0.001$). This pattern was also observed in the CS group, where CRP levels ≥ 3 mg/L showed a worse lipid profile and a higher score of the cardiometabolic indexes than subjects with CRP levels < 3 mg/L (Table 2).

Table 2. Biochemical and cardiometabolic status stratified according to CVD risk by CRP in SLE patients and CS.

Variable	CVD Risk by CRP in SLE Patients				CVD Risk by CRP in CS			
	Low Risk (<1 mg/L) n = 30	Average Risk (≥1 to <3 mg/L) n = 33	High Risk (≥3 mg/L) n = 113	p Value	Low Risk (<1 mg/L) n = 84	Average Risk (≥1 to <3 mg/L) n = 46	High Risk (≥3 mg/L) n = 45	p Value
Glucose (mg/L) [a]	85.9 (76.1–154)	86 (65–116)	89 (70–133)	0.71	84.9 (72.9–98.9)	86 (75.1–105.1)	96.1 (82.2–174.8)	0.001
Triglycerides (mg/L) [a]	112 (45–214)	83 (47–287)	124 (61–245.7)	<0.001	65.6 (36–135.3)	76.1 (45.8–170.1)	109.3 (49.7–225.2)	<0.001
Total cholesterol (mg/L) [a]	163 (110.7–251)	159 (109–260)	171 (119.5–249.5)	0.25	162.7 (123.6–228.6)	169.2 (118.8–229.9)	190 (131.7–274)	0.01
LDL-C (mg/L) [a]	84.7 (53.2–128.7)	89.5 (53.6–172)	72.3 (41.3–138.1)	0.03	92 (59–157.2)	96 (55–147.2)	110.7 (63.1–180.2)	<0.01
HDL-C (mg/L) [a]	41.3 (19.1–71.6)	45.4 (21.7–71.2)	26.2 (12.8–62.7)	<0.001	54.6 (40.3–83)	50.4 (32.6–70.6)	45.5 (31.7–66.4)	<0.001
Castelli index (TC/HDL-C) [a]	3.7 (2.4–10.8)	3.7 (2.2–8.4)	6.5 (2.8–14.9)	<0.001	2.8 (2.1–4.9)	3.2 (2.4–6.5)	4.3 (2.3–6.3)	<0.001
Castelli CVD risk % (n) [b]								
Low risk (<4.5)	78.6 (22/28)	70 (23/33)	36 (37/104)	<0.001	90.5 (76/84)	73.9 (34/46)	53.3 (24/45)	<0.001
Moderate risk (≥4.5 to <7.0)	10.7 (3/28)	24 (8/33)	16.3 (17/104)		8.3 (7/84)	21.7 (10/46)	46.7 (21/45)	
High risk (≥7.0)	10.7 (3/28)	6 (2/33)	48 (50/104)		1.2 (1/84)	4.4 (2/46)	0 (0/45)	
Kannel Index (LDL-C/HDL-C) [a]	1.8 (1–4.4)	2 (1.1–3.4)	2.5 (1.2–6.3)	<0.001	1.7 (0.86–3.2)	1.8 (1.1–3.5)	2.5 (1.2–3.8)	<0.001
Kannel CVD risk % (n) [b]								
Low risk (<3)	82.1 (23/28)	87.9 (29/33)	59.6 (62/104)	0.001	93 (78/84)	84.4 (38/45)	66.7 (30/45)	0.001
High risk (≥3)	17.9 (5/28)	12.1 (4/33)	40.4 (42/104)		7 (6/84)	15.6 (7/45)	33.3 (15/45)	
Triglycerides/HDL-C ratio	1.9 (1.1–9.3)	2.1 (0.8–5.6)	4.4 (1.3–15)	<0.001	1.2 (0.4–2.8)	1.4 (0.7–5)	2.5 (0.8–5.8)	<0.001
Triglycerides/HDL-C risk % (n) [b]								
Low risk (<3)	68 (19/28)	76 (25/33)	29 (30/104)	<0.001	96.4 (81/84)	80.4 (37/46)	58 (26/45)	<0.001
High risk (≥3)	32 (9/28)	24 (8/33)	71 (74/104)		3.6 (3/84)	19.6 (9/46)	42 (19/45)	
LAP (score) [a]	25 (4.2–72.5)	26.1 (7.7–86)	41.7 (7.6–95.2)	0.02	8.9 (1.5–38.3)	18.9 (4.4–59.7)	41.8 (5.5–106.2)	<0.001
CMI (score) [a]	1 (0.4–3.5)	1.1 (0.4–3)	1.4 (0.4–3.3)	0.03	0.5 (0.19–2.4)	0.8 (0.3–2.9)	1.2 (0.4–10)	<0.001

[a] Data provided in median (percentile: p5th–p95th), p value: Kruskal–Wallis test. [b] Data provided in percentages (n). The bold numbers indicate variables with significant differences. **SLE:** systemic lupus erythematosus patients; **CS:** control subjects; **HDL-C:** high-density lipoprotein cholesterol; **CVD:** cardiovascular disease; **TC:** total cholesterol; **LAP:** lipid accumulation products; LAP = (waist in cm − 58)*(triglycerides mmol/L); **CMI:** cardiometabolic index; CMI = (triglycerides/HDL-C). p value: Pearson χ^2 test. **LDL-C:** low-density lipoprotein cholesterol;

Additionally, we stratified the complement C3 and C4 serum levels according to cardiovascular risk by CRP, and we did not observe significant differences in C3 according to CRP levels, but we found a tendency for lower C4 levels in SLE patients with average ($\geq$1 mg/L) and high cardiovascular risk ($\geq$3 mg/L) compared to SLE patients with low risk (<1 mg/L) (CRP low risk: 25.2 mg/dL; average risk: 12.5 mg/dL; high risk: 15.5 mg/dL; $p = 0.06$). Regarding the SLE treatment, patients with CQ treatment had higher CRP serum levels than SLE patients with HCQ treatment (CQ = 5 mg/L vs. HCQ = 1.7 mg/L; $p < 0.001$). According to the classification for CVD risk by CRP, a high CVD risk was observed in SLE patients with CQ treatment vs. HCQ treatment (CQ = 77.2% vs. HCQ = 22.8%; $p < 0.001$). A similar pattern was observed in SLE patients who received prednisone treatment, presenting higher CRP serum levels (with prednisone = 5.7 mg/L vs. without prednisone = 2.6 mg/L; $p < 0.001$) and a higher frequency of high CVD risk evaluated by CRP in comparison to SLE patients without prednisone treatment (with prednisone = 64.6% vs. without prednisone = 35.4%; $p < 0.001$).

Based on the previous results, we determined the correlation between body composition and cardiometabolic status with CRP levels. In all the participants we found a significant correlation between CRP levels and all the body composition and cardiometabolic variables evaluated, except total cholesterol. In the SLE group, the CRP levels positively correlated with body composition variables such as weight (r = 0.22; $p < 0.01$), BMI (r = 0.28 $p < 0.001$), WHtR (r = 0.21; $p = 0.03$) and fat mass (r = 0.21; $p = 0.03$). In the CS group, weight (r = 0.56; $p < 0.001$), waist (r = 0.60; $p < 0.001$), BMI (r = 0.63; $p < 0.001$), WHR score (r = 0.45; $p < 0.001$), WHtR score (r = 0.59; $p < 0.001$) and fat mass (r = 65; $p < 0.001$) correlated positively, while muscle mass (r = -0.61; $p < 0.001$), and body water (r = -0.65; $p < 0.001$) were negatively correlated with CRP levels (Table 3).

Table 3. Correlations between body composition, cardiometabolic status, and SLE clinical features with CRP in both study groups.

Variables	All Participants CRP (mg/L)		SLE Patients CRP (mg/L)		CS CRP (mg/L)	
	* r	p Value	* r	p Value	* r	p Value
Body composition						
Weight (kg)	0.44	<0.001	0.22	<0.01	0.56	<0.001
Waist (cm)	0.52	<0.001	0.19	0.05	0.60	<0.001
BMI (kg/m^2)	0.52	<0.001	0.28	<0.001	0.63	<0.001
WHR (score)	0.42	<0.001	0.11	0.24	0.45	<0.001
WHtR (score)	0.53	<0.001	0.21	0.03	0.59	<0.001
Fat mass (%)	0.50	<0.001	0.21	0.03	0.65	<0.001
Muscle mass (kg)	-0.48	<0.001	-0.17	0.08	-0.61	<0.001
Body water (%)	-0.51	<0.001	-0.17	0.08	-0.65	<0.001
Cardiometabolic status						
Glucose (mg/L)	0.22	<0.001	0.08	0.29	0.39	<0.001
Triglycerides (mg/L)	0.42	<0.001	0.18	0.01	0.42	<0.001
Total cholesterol (mg/L)	0.07	0.15	0.01	0.84	0.20	<0.01
LDL-C (mg/L)	-0.13	0.01	-0.24	0.001	0.21	<0.01
HDL-C (mg/L)	-0.44	<0.001	-0.37	<0.001	-0.31	<0.001
Castelli index (TC/HDL-C)	0.47	<0.001	0.35	<0.001	0.40	<0.001
Kannel Index (LDL-C/HDL-C)	0.36	<0.001	0.23	<0.01	0.36	<0.001
Triglycerides/HDL-C ratio (score)	0.52	<0.001	0.38	<0.001	0.45	<0.001
LAP (score)	0.51	<0.001	0.18	0.06	0.59	<0.001
CMI (score)	0.46	<0.001	0.21	0.03	0.51	<0.001
SLE clinical features						
Mex-SLEDAI (score)	-	-	0.22	<0.01	-	-
Disease duration (years)	-	-	0.20	<0.01	-	-

* Spearman correlation test. The bold numbers indicate variables with significant differences. **SLE:** systemic lupus erythematosus; **CS:** control subjects; **CRP:** C-reactive protein; **BMI:** body mass index; **WHR:** waist to hip ratio; **WHtR:** waist to height ratio (cm/cm); **LDL-C:** low-density lipoprotein cholesterol; **HDL-C:** high-density lipoprotein cholesterol; **TC:** total cholesterol; **LAP:** lipid accumulation products; LAP = (waist in cm $-$ 58)*(triglycerides mmol/L); **CMI:** cardiometabolic index; CMI = (triglycerides/HDL-C).

Regarding cardiometabolic status, in SLE patients we observed a positive correlation between triglycerides levels (r = 0.18; p = 0.01), the Castelli index (r = 0.35; p < 0.001), the Kannel index (r = 0.23; p < 0.01), the triglycerides-HDL-C ratio (r = 0.38; p < 0.001), and CMI score (r = 0.21; p = 0.03), and a negative correlation between LDL-C (r = −0.24; p = 0.001), and HDL-C (r = −0.37; p < 0.001) with CRP levels. Moderate correlations were observed in the CS group between CRP levels and the cardiometabolic variables. Regarding SLE patients, the CRP levels correlated positively with the Mex-SLEDAI score (r = 0.22; p < 0.01) and with disease duration (r = 0.20; p < 0.01) (Table 3).

3.4. Association of CRP Levels with Cardiometabolic Variables and Clinical Disease Activity

We analyzed the association of the high cardiovascular risk by CRP levels (≥3 mg/L) with cardiometabolic variables and clinical disease activity in SLE patients by logistic regression models. We found that SLE patients with CRP levels ≥ 3 mg/L had a significantly higher risk of presenting clinical disease activity with a Mex-SLEDAI ≥ 2 (OR = 2.5; CI = 1.03–6.2; p = 0.04), higher risk of having a high LAP score ≥ Tertile 3rd (OR = 3.01; CI = 1.04–8.7; p = 0.04), higher risk of a triglycerides/HDL-C index score ≥ 3 (OR = 5.2; IC = 2.1–12.8; p < 0.001), Kannel index score ≥ 3 (OR = 3.1; IC = 1.1–8.1; p = 0.03), and Castelli index score ≥ 7 (OR = 6.6; IC = 2.5–17.8; p < 0.001) in comparison with SLE patients with CRP < 1 mg/L (Figure 2).

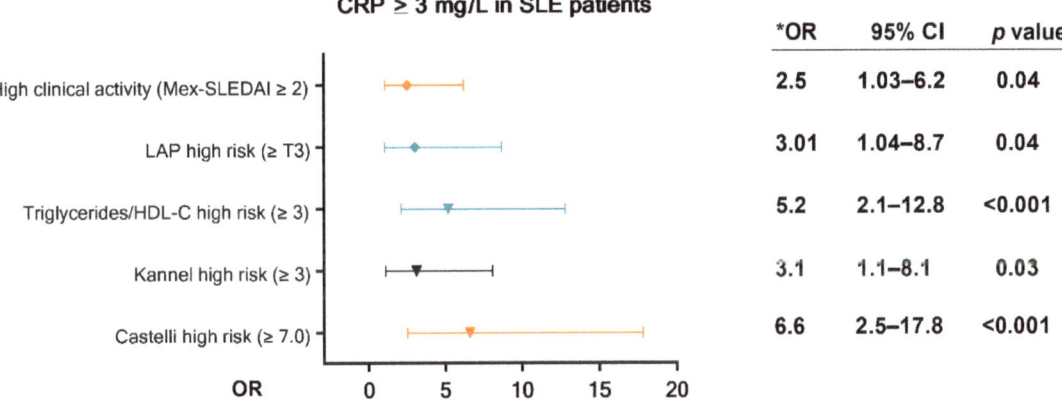

Figure 2. Association of the CRP levels (≥3 mg/L) with clinical activity and cardiometabolic variables in SLE. Castelli index: total cholesterol/HDL-C; Kannel index: LDL-C/HDL-C ratio; LAP score: (waist circumference, cm–58) (TG, mmol/L). T3: ≥31.06 to maximum value; OR: odds ratio, confidence interval 95%, p values < 0.05. * Reference group: SLE patients with CRP < 1 mg/L.

Finally, based on the previous results, we determined in a linear regression model that the high CRP levels (≥3 mg/L) increased 6.1 points of the Mex-SLEDAI score when we adjusted the model for fat mass percentage (β coefficient = 6.1; IC = 2.8–9.1; R^2 = 0.14; p <0.001). These findings suggest that the association found between CRP and the clinical activity is not influenced by fat mass. When we adjusted by other variables such as BMI, age, and fat mass percentage, the significant association remained (β coefficient = 5.8; IC = 2.5–9.4; R^2 = 0.15; p = 0.001), which demonstrates that the associations found between CRP and clinical disease activity were independent of these variables that could influence the CRP serum levels.

4. Discussion

In this present study, we found that SLE patients had excess weight and altered waist circumference related to CVD risk. Previous studies conducted on SLE populations supported these findings; the SLE patients showed a high frequency of excess weight associated with cardiovascular disease risk factors [24,25]. SLE patients also showed higher triglycerides and lower HDL-C levels compared to CS. These findings are in accordance with the classical "lupus lipoprotein pattern", characterized by high triglycerides and low HDL-C but unchanged LDL-C. In this pattern, there is also the presence of some autoantibodies such as anti-HDL-C and anti-lipoprotein lipase [26]; however, the lipid autoantibodies were not evaluated in this study.

Notably, we found that SLE patients had a high cardiovascular risk determined by cardiometabolic indexes such as the Castelli index, Kannel index, triglycerides/HDL-C ratio, CMI index, and LAP index. The worse cardiometabolic status in SLE than CS can be partly explained by the high frequency of traditional risk factors such as diabetes mellitus, hypertension, central obesity, dyslipidemia, and pharmacotherapy such as glucocorticoids in these patients. Previous studies have reported rates of dyslipidemia in SLE patients ranging from 36% at the time of diagnosis to more than 60% within a three-year follow up [27]. Additionally, SLE treatment plays a relevant role in developing CVD in these patients. Prednisone use has been associated with an altered lipoprotein profile that could be a potential mechanism for the enhanced atherogenic risk in SLE. Immunological mechanisms have also been related to the development of atherosclerosis in SLE, an imbalance between endothelial damage and atheroprotective mechanisms and autoantibodies such as anti-endothelial cell (AEC) and anti-oxLDL could participate in the cardiovascular disturbances in SLE [28].

CRP is accepted as an independent risk factor for cardiovascular events in the general population [29]. It is one of the components of the Reynolds cardiovascular risk score [30], but its role in CVD and SLE is still controversial; based on previous findings, we assessed the relationship of CRP with biochemical and cardiometabolic variables. According to this, SLE patients with high cardiovascular risk assessed by CRP (≥ 3 mg/L) showed significantly higher triglyceride levels and lower HDL-C levels than patients at low and average risk. Patients with high CRP levels (≥ 3 mg/L) also presented higher scores with regard to the Castelli, Kannel, triglycerides/HDL-C, LAP, and CMI indices. Differences according to CRP levels were also observed in the CS group; these results suggest that CRP could determine cardiovascular status in an indirect way through influencing cardiometabolic variables.

Following these reported findings, we found a positive correlation between CRP levels and anthropometric variables such as weight, waist, BMI, WHR, and fat mass percentage. Previous cross-sectional studies have shown that CRP correlates with obesity indicators such as BMI, WHR, and adiposity [31,32]; some authors even suggest that the fat mass has a greater ability to classify subjects with high CRP serum levels compared with BMI and WHR [32]. The mechanism linked to CRP and fat mass could be mediated by adipose tissue, which is the main source of inflammatory cytokines; approximately 30% of total IL-6 production may arise in adipose tissue; this interleukin is the main stimulant for CRP production [33].

CRP levels are also positively correlated with biochemical variables such as triglycerides and the Castelli, Kannel, CMI, and triglycerides/HDL-C cardiometabolic indexes, and negatively correlated with HDL-C levels. Our results agree with previous studies conducted on SLE populations that reported a correlation between CRP levels and lipid profile alterations, diabetes, obesity, and BMI. They also found that triglyceride levels and the triglycerides/HDL-C ratio positively correlated with CRP levels [11].

The relationship between CRP and dyslipidemia could be explained by excessive lipids accumulating in the arterial wall, inducing an inflammatory response; it accelerates lipid deposition and amplifies the inflammation producing inflammatory factors such as CRP [34]. CRP can bind to LDL-C in atherosclerotic plaques, leading to complement activation, and promoting inflammation and atherosclerosis. Pan He et al. reported that CRP plays a mediator role in the relationship between dyslipidemia and coronary arterial disease [34]. On the other hand, in normal conditions HDL-C promotes reverse cholesterol transport and inhibits LDL-C oxidation; however, under inflammatory conditions characterized by high levels of inflammatory markers such as IL-6, the antioxidant and anti-atherogenic capacity of HDL-C may be lower. Additionally, the inflammatory process could alter LPL activity, resulting in the accumulation of VLDL, thereby increasing triglycerides and lowering the HDL-C serum levels [4]. However, to our knowledge, the exact mechanism through which CRP affects lipid metabolism is still unclear.

Concerning CRP levels in SLE compared to general populations, some studies have reported no differences in CRP levels between SLE patients vs. the general population. Controversial results have been reported, where SLE patients used to have lower CRP levels than healthy subjects [35]. The mechanism suggested in other studies to alter and cause inhomogeneous levels of CRP in SLE patients are the lower CRP production through the increased production of IFN-α, which is characteristic in active SLE. This event is brought about via the enhancer binding protein (C/EBPs) and STAT3, affecting the inhibition of CRP production [35].

Conversely, we found that SLE patients have higher CRP levels than healthy individuals. These findings also are in accordance with other studies conducted on different SLE populations [10,12]. We also showed that CRP levels had a high capacity to discriminate between SLE and CS using ROC curves. According to this, the inconsistencies reported in the literature could be derived from the method used to determine CRP levels; conventional methods can only detect values above 3 mg/L, while CRP can detect at a level as low as 0.3 mg/L [36]. On the other hand, polymorphisms in *the CRP* gene could alter *CRP* transcription or mRNA stability depending on its location, which could increase CRP levels, according to some studies conducted on the Mexican population [37,38]. A study conducted on SLE patients from Brazil showed an association between rs1130864 *CRP* polymorphism and SLE susceptibility [39], while Enocsson et al. reported that IFN-α downregulates CRP expression, and the rs1205 *CRP* polymorphism could explain the low basal CRP and the inadequate CRP responses among active SLE patients [40]. However, it is well known that there are racial and ethnic disparities in the allele frequency distribution of *CRP* polymorphisms [41], which could explain in part the discrepancies reported in the literature about the association of *CRP* polymorphism with genetic risk and the clinical disease activity in SLE populations with different genetic backgrounds.

The immunomodulatory role of CRP is widely described; it could exert inflammatory and anti-inflammatory activities by regulating complement activation through the binding of factor H, promoting the binding of the apoptotic materials and their clearance [36]. We showed that there are no differences in C3 complement levels according to CRP stratification, but SLE patients with average and high CVD risk by CRP levels (≥ 1 mg/L) tended to have lower C4 complement levels than patients with low CRP levels (<1 mg/L). A study conducted on SLE patients from China reported a negative correlation between C3 and C4 complement levels and the clinical disease activity; however, CRP serum levels were not associated with clinical disease activity [42].

The role of CRP in clinical disease activity in SLE is still complex and controversial; some studies reported that CRP levels are normal or only modestly elevated in active SLE and that there is no relationship between CRP levels and clinical disease activity [12,13]. In contrast, we found that patients with active SLE had higher CRP levels than inactive SLE patients; additionally, we observed a positive correlation between Mex-SLEDAI score and CRP levels when we adjusted for some variables that could influence it, such as age, fat mass, and BMI [32]. It has been reported that acute phase reactants such as CRP tend to increase with age [43]. Notably, we observed that the association between CRP levels and clinical disease activity in SLE is independent of this factor. Concerning fat mass and BMI, a previous study conducted on our SLE population reported that patients with excess weight (BMI ≥ 25 kg/m^2) had high clinical disease activity. Additionally, a positive correlation between Mex-SLEDAI score and BMI was observed [44]. According to this, we observed that the relationship between CRP levels and clinical disease activity is also independent of the excess weight. Mok et al. reported that CRP levels were detectable in 77% of SLE patients, and CRP correlated with SLEDAI scores in SLE patients from USA [36]. Another study conducted on SLE patients from Spain also showed a significant correlation between CRP levels and the clinical disease activity assessed by the SLEDAI-2K score [11].

The discrepancies reported about CRP and clinical disease activity in SLE in different studies could be related to its structure; it has been reported that two structures of CRP exist: the pentameric (pCRP) and monomeric CRP (mCRP) forms. These exert different biological functions. pCRP binds and opsonizes dying cells and cell remnants, facilitating phagocytosis via Fc-receptor binding [7,45]. The mCRP form is an efficient activator of the classical complement pathway involving C1, C2, C3, and C4 complement fractions, acting as a regulator of the alternative complement pathway. mCRP is considered a more pro-inflammatory form, and could promote the differentiation of monocytes toward a pro-inflammatory M1 phenotype [46], resulting in a high secretion of inflammatory cytokines such as IL-6 and IL-1 [47]; this, in a feedback loop, induces CRP synthesis in hepatocytes at the transcriptional level through STAT3 activation [48]. Additionally, mCRP rather than pCRP has been related to cardiovascular disturbances [46]; previously, it was reported that the high cardiovascular risk determined by biochemical variables and cardiometabolic indexes in SLE patients was associated with clinical disease activity [14]. Based on this, we hypothesized that the relationship between CRP and active SLE could increase cardiovascular risk and subsequently increase the inflammatory process and clinical activity.

In other pathologies such as cancer, the roles of pCRP and mCRP have also been described [49]. However, neither study conducted on SLE patients have reported the role of CRP according to its structure. pCRP's structure is dependent upon the presence of calcium ions. The binding of pCRP to a damaged cell membrane, inflammatory conditions, and oxidative stress promote conformational switching from pCRP to mCRP [7]. To date, no studies have measured the conversion rate from pCRP to mCRP in SLE, and if there is a differential relationship according to CRP structure with CVD risk and clinical disease activity. In our study, we observed that the high serum levels of CRP ($\geq$3 mg/L) were associated with high clinical activity in SLE. We also showed that SLE patients with CRP levels $\geq$ 3 mg/L had a high chance of being at high cardiometabolic risk, assessed by the LAP, Castelli, triglycerides/HDL-C, and Kannel indexes. Based on these results, we suggest that CRP levels could be an additional biomarker to monitor cardiometabolic risk and the clinical disease activity in SLE; however, further studies are necessary to support these findings. Additionally, CRP could be a useful target to reduce CVD risk and the clinical disease activity in SLE. In populations with cardiovascular events, the CRP apheresis technique showed to be promising for decreasing CRP levels [9], and this technique could be applied to SLE patients with CRP-mediated inflammatory conditions.

Despite its strengths, this study had limitations: first, our comparative cross-sectional design is limited by merely showing a relationship between the CRP levels, cardiometabolic status, and clinical disease activity; however, we do not suggest causality because it only provides information on a specific point in time. Second, another limitation is that some SLE patients evaluated had incomplete clinical, biochemical, and pharmacotherapy administered data that we could not retrieve from the patient's medical records or at the time of quantifying the analytes presented in this study. Third, we were not able to assess IL-6 serum levels, which is responsible for stimulating CRP production. Finally, we only provided information about the global clinical disease activity and renal activity in our population; however, we were not able to assess the clinical activity of other organs such as the skin, joints, pleura, or central nervous system. Despite its weaknesses, the present study provides evidence of the association between high CRP levels with high cardiometabolic risk and clinical disease activity in SLE patients.

Further prospective studies on SLE Mexican population cohorts are needed to be performed to evaluate causality in the relationship of CRP serum levels with cardiometabolic and organ-specific disease activity outcomes. Moreover, it will be necessary to evaluate the specific pathogenic role of the monomeric or pentameric CRP structures in autoimmune conditions, as well as the potential correlation between CRP, IL-6, and other pro-inflammatory cytokines in SLE. Finally, we need to determine the influence of some genetic variants in the CRP gene and the possible epigenetic interactions with genes involved in CRP synthesis.

5. Conclusions

The present study provides evidence of the association between high CRP levels with high cardiometabolic risk in SLE patients and the general population. Notably, in SLE patients, CRP serum levels were also associated with clinical disease activity. Therefore, CRP could be an additional biomarker to monitor cardiometabolic risk and clinical disease activity in SLE.

Author Contributions: Conceptualization, U.d.l.C.-M.; Data curation, P.E.M.-G., A.I.R.-B., M.R.M.-M., B.C.-L. and M.R.-E.; Formal analysis, K.P.-C., I.P.-R., M.M.-B., A.I.R.-B., M.R.M.-M., B.C.-L., M.R.-E., B.V.-L., S.C.-C. and U.d.l.C.-M.; Funding acquisition, U.d.l.C.-M.; Investigation, K.P.-C., P.E.M.-G., A.I.R.-B., M.R.M.-M., B.C.-L., M.R.-E. and S.C.-C.; Methodology, I.P.-R., M.M.-B., B.V.-L. and U.d.l.C.-M.; Project administration, U.d.l.C.-M.; Writing—original draft, K.P.-C.; Writing—review and editing, K.P.-C., I.P.-R., P.E.M.-G., M.M.-B., B.V.-L., S.C.-C. and U.d.l.C.-M. All authors have read and agreed to the published version of the manuscript.

Funding: This study was supported by Grant No. UDG-PTC 1401 for Ulises de la Cruz-Mosso, PhD (U.D.C.M.), from the Programa de Apoyo a la Mejora en las Condiciones de Producción de los Miembros del SNI y SNCA 2019-2021 (U.d.l.C.-M.) from the University of Guadalajara. The funding source was not involved in any step of the study.

Institutional Review Board Statement: This study was conducted in accordance with the Declaration of Helsinki and approved by the Institutional Research Ethical Committee of the University of Guadalajara (CI-05018 CUCS-UdeG), based on national and international ethical guidelines.

Informed Consent Statement: All SLE patients and CS before enrollment to the study provided signed written informed consent according to the ethical guidelines.

Data Availability Statement: Data used to support the findings of this study are available from the corresponding author upon reasonable request.

Acknowledgments: We acknowledge the clinical and logistic support for the recruitment of the SLE patients given by the Rheumatologists Sergio Cerpa-Cruz, and Gloria Esther Martínez Bonilla, from the Departamento de Reumatología, O.P.D. Hospital Civil de Guadalajara Fray Antonio Alcalde, Guadalajara, Jalisco, Mexico.

Conflicts of Interest: The authors declare no conflict of interest and the funders had no role in the design of the study; in the collection, analyses, or interpretation of data; in the writing of the manuscript, or in the decision to publish the results.

References

1. Ye, Y.; Wu, T.; Zhang, T.; Han, J.; Habazi, D.; Saxena, R.; Mohan, C. Elevated oxidized lipids, anti-lipid autoantibodies and oxidized lipid immune complexes in active SLE. *Clin. Immunol.* **2019**, *205*, 43–48. [CrossRef] [PubMed]
2. Pan, L.; Lu, M.-P.; Wang, J.-H.; Xu, M.; Yang, S.-R. Immunological pathogenesis and treatment of systemic lupus erythematosus. *World J. Pediatr.* **2020**, *16*, 19–30. [CrossRef] [PubMed]
3. Urowitz, M.B. The Bimodal Mortality Pattern of Systemic Lupus Erythematosus. Systemic Lupus Erythematosus. *Am. J. Med.* **1976**, *5*, 221–225. [CrossRef]
4. Szabó, M.Z.; Szodoray, P.; Kiss, E. Dyslipidemia in systemic lupus erythematosus. *Immunol. Res.* **2017**, *65*, 543–550. [CrossRef]
5. Lin, C.-Y.; Shih, C.-C.; Yeh, C.-C.; Chou, W.-H.; Chen, T.-L.; Liao, C.-C. Increased risk of acute myocardial infarction and mortality in patients with systemic lupus erythematosus: Two nationwide retrospective cohort studies. *Int. J. Cardiol.* **2014**, *176*, 847–851. [CrossRef]
6. Sinicato, N.A. Risk Factors in Cardiovascular Disease in Systemic Lupus Erythematosus. *Curr. Cardiol.* **2013**, *5*, 15–19.
7. Enocsson, H.; Karlsson, J.; Li, H.-Y.; Wu, Y.; Kushner, I.; Wetterö, J.; Sjöwall, C. The Complex Role of C-Reactive Protein in Systemic Lupus Erythematosus. *J. Clin. Med.* **2021**, *10*, 5837. [CrossRef]
8. Boncler, M.; Wu, Y.; Watala, C. The Multiple Faces of C-Reactive Protein—Physiological and Pathophysiological Implications in Cardiovascular Disease. *Molecules* **2019**, *24*, 2062. [CrossRef]
9. Kayser, S.; Brunner, P.; Althaus, K.; Dorst, J.; Sheriff, A. Selective Apheresis of C-Reactive Protein for Treatment of Indications with Elevated CRP Concentrations. *J. Clin. Med.* **2020**, *9*, 2947. [CrossRef]

10. Salomão, R.G.; de Carvalho, L.M.; Izumi, C.; Czernisz, É.S.; Rosa, J.C.; Antonini, S.R.R.; Bueno, A.C.; do Vale Almada, M.O.R.; de Almeida Coelho-Landell, C.; Jordão, A.A.; et al. Homocysteine, folate, hs-C-reactive protein, tumor necrosis factor alpha and inflammatory proteins: Are these biomarkers related to nutritional status and cardiovascular risk in childhood-onset systemic lupus erythematosus? *Pediatr. Rheumatol. Online J.* **2018**, *16*, 4. [CrossRef]
11. Pocovi-Gerardino, G.; Correa-Rodríguez, M.; Rubio, J.-L.C.; Fernández, R.R.; Amada, M.M.; Caparros, M.-G.C.; Rueda-Medina, B.; Ortego-Centeno, N. The Relationships of High-Sensitivity C-Reactive Protein and Homocysteine Levels with Disease Activity, Damage Accrual, and Cardiovascular Risk in Systemic Lupus Erythematosus. *Biol. Res. Nurs.* **2020**, *22*, 169–177. [CrossRef]
12. Barnes, E.V.; Narain, S.; Naranjo, A.; Shuster, J.; Segal, M.S.; Sobel, E.S.; Armstrong, A.E.; Santiago, B.E.; Reeves, W.H.; Richards, H.B. High sensitivity C-reactive protein in systemic lupus erythematosus: Relation to disease activity, clinical presentation and implications for cardiovascular risk. *Lupus* **2005**, *14*, 576–582. [CrossRef] [PubMed]
13. Luo, K.-L.; Yang, Y.-H.; Lin, Y.-T.; Hu, Y.-C.; Yu, H.-H.; Wang, L.-C.; Chiang, B.-L.; Lee, J.-H. Differential parameters between activity flare and acute infection in pediatric patients with systemic lupus erythematosus. *Sci. Rep.* **2020**, *10*, 19913. [CrossRef] [PubMed]
14. Campos-López, B.; Meza-Meza, M.R.; Parra-Rojas, I.; Ruiz-Ballesteros, A.I.; Vizmanos-Lamotte, B.; Muñoz-Valle, J.F.; Montoya-Buelna, M.; Cerpa-Cruz, S.; Bernal-Hernández, L.E.; De la Cruz-Mosso, U. Association of cardiometabolic risk status with clinical activity and damage in systemic lupus erythematosus patients: A cross-sectional study. *Clin. Immunol.* **2021**, *222*, 108637. [CrossRef] [PubMed]
15. Hochberg, M.C. Updating the American college of rheumatology revised criteria for the classification of systemic lupus erythematosus. *Arthritis Rheum.* **1997**, *40*, 1725. [CrossRef]
16. Uribe, A.G.; Vilá, L.M.; McGwin, G., Jr.; Sanchez, M.L.; Reveille, J.D.; Alarcón, G.S. The Systemic Lupus Activity Measure-Revised, the Mexican Systemic Lupus Erythematosus Disease Activity Index (SLEDAI), and a Modified SLEDAI-2K Are Adequate Instruments to Measure Disease Activity in Systemic Lupus Erythematosus. *J. Rheumatol.* **2004**, *10*, 1934–1940.
17. World Health Organization. *Waist Circumference and Waist-Hip Ratio: Report of a WHO Expert Consultation, Geneva, 8–11 December 2008*; World Health Organization: Geneva, Switzerland, 2011.
18. World Health Organization. Regional Office for the Eastern Mediterranean. In *List of Basic Sources in English for a Medical Faculty Library*; World Health Organization: Geneva, Switzerland, 2010.
19. Ashwell, M.; Gunn, P.; Gibson, S. Waist-to-height ratio is a better screening tool than waist circumference and BMI for adult cardiometabolic risk factors: Systematic review and meta-analysis: Waist-to-height ratio as a screening tool. *Obes. Rev.* **2012**, *13*, 275–286. [CrossRef]
20. Wakabayashi, I.; Daimon, T. The "cardiometabolic index" as a new marker determined by adiposity and blood lipids for discrimination of diabetes mellitus. *Clin. Chim. Acta* **2015**, *438*, 274–278. [CrossRef]
21. Pearson, T.A.; Mensah, G.A.; Alexander, R.W.; Anderson, J.L.; Cannon, R.O.; Criqui, M.; Fadl, Y.Y.; Fortmann, S.P.; Hong, Y.; Myers, G.L.; et al. Markers of Inflammation and Cardiovascular Disease: Application to Clinical and Public Health Practice: A Statement for Healthcare Professionals from the Centers for Disease Control and Prevention and the American Heart Association. *Circ. J.* **2003**, *107*, 499–511. [CrossRef]
22. Ricardo-Navarro Vargas, J.; Matiz-Camacho, H.; Osorio-Esquivel, J. Evidence-based clinical practice manual: Cardiopulmonary-cerebral resuscitation. *Rev. Colom. Anestesiol.* **2015**, *43*, 9–19. [CrossRef]
23. Kahn, H.S. The «lipid accumulation product» performs better than the body mass index for recognizing cardiovascular risk: A population-based comparison. *BMC Cardiovasc. Disord.* **2005**, *5*, 26. [CrossRef] [PubMed]
24. de Miranda Moura dos Santos, F.; Borges, M.C.; Telles, R.W.; Correia, M.I.T.D.; Lanna, C.C.D. Excess weight and associated risk factors in patients with systemic lupus erythematosus. *Rheumatol. Int.* **2013**, *33*, 681–688. [CrossRef] [PubMed]
25. Rizk, A.; Gheita, T.A.; Nassef, S.; Abdallah, A. The impact of obesity in systemic lupus erythematosus on disease parameters, quality of life, functional capacity and the risk of atherosclerosis: Obesity in SLE. *Int. J. Rheum Dis.* **2012**, *15*, 261–267. [CrossRef] [PubMed]
26. Hua, X.; Su, J.; Svenungsson, E.; Hurt-Camejo, E.; Jensen-Urstad, K.; Angelin, B.; Båvenholm, P.; Frostegård, J. Dyslipidaemia and lipoprotein pattern in systemic lupus erythematosus (SLE) and SLE-related cardiovascular disease. *Scand. J. Rheumatol.* **2009**, *38*, 184–189. [CrossRef] [PubMed]
27. Urowitz, M.B.; Gladman, D.; Ibañez, D.; Fortin, P.; Sanchez-Guerrero, J.; Bae, S.; Clarke, A.; Bernatsky, S.; Gordon, C.; Hanly, J.; et al. Accumulation of coronary artery disease risk factors over three years: Data from an international inception cohort. *Arthritis Rheum.* **2008**, *59*, 176–180. [CrossRef] [PubMed]
28. Giannelou, M.; Mavragani, C.P. Cardiovascular disease in systemic lupus erythematosus: A comprehensive update. *J. Autoimmun.* **2017**, *82*, 1–12. [CrossRef]
29. Stephen, K.; Emmanuele, D.; Gordon, L.; Mark, B.; Simon, G.; Rory, C.; Jonh, D.; Emerging Risk Factors Collaboration. C-reactive protein concentration and risk of coronary heart disease, stroke, and mortality: An individual participant meta-analysis. *Lancet* **2010**, *375*, 9.
30. Ridker, P.M.; Buring, J.E.; Rifai, N.; Cook, N.R. Development and Validation of Improved Algorithms for the Assessment of Global Cardiovascular Risk in Women: The Reynolds Risk Score. *JAMA* **2007**, *297*, 611. [CrossRef]

31. Fröhlich, M.; Imhof, A.; Berg, G.; Hutchinson, W.L.; Pepys, M.B.; Boeing, H.; Muche, R.; Brenner, H.; Koenig, W. Association between C-reactive protein and features of the metabolic syndrome: A population-based study. *Diabetes Care* **2000**, *23*, 1835–1839. [CrossRef]
32. Lin, C.-C.; Kardia, S.L.; Li, C.-I.; Liu, C.-S.; Lai, M.-M.; Lin, W.-Y.; Chang, P.-C.; Lee, Y.-D.; Chen, C.-C.; Lin, C.-H.; et al. The relationship of high sensitivity C-reactive protein to percent body fat mass, body mass index, waist-to-hip ratio, and waist circumference in a Taiwanese population. *BMC Public Health* **2010**, *10*, 579. [CrossRef]
33. Mohamed-Ali, V. Subcutaneous Adipose Tissue Releases Interleukin-6, But Not Tumor Necrosis Factor-Alpha, in Vivo. *J. Clin. Endocrinol. Metab.* **1997**, *82*, 4196–4200. [PubMed]
34. He, P.; Fan, S.; Guan, J.; Song, W.; Obore, N.; Chen, W.; Zhi, H.; Wang, L. Mediation analysis for the relationship between dyslipidemia and coronary artery disease via hypersensitive C-reactive protein in a case-control study. *Coron. Artery Dis.* **2020**, *31*, 613–619. [CrossRef] [PubMed]
35. Meyer, O. Anti-CRP antibodies in systemic lupus erythematosus. *Jt. Bone Spine.* **2010**, *77*, 384–389. [CrossRef] [PubMed]
36. Mok, C.C.; Birmingham, D.J.; Ho, L.Y.; Hebert, L.A.; Rovin, B.H. High-sensitivity C-reactive protein, disease activity, and cardiovascular risk factors in systemic lupus erythematosus. *Arthritis Care Res.* **2013**, *65*, 441–447. [CrossRef] [PubMed]
37. Martínez-Calleja, A.; Quiróz-Vargas, I.; Parra-Rojas, I.; Muñoz-Valle, J.F.; Leyva-Vázquez, M.A.; Fernández-Tilapa, G.; Vences-Velázquez, A.; Cruz, M.; Salazar-Martínez, E.; Flores-Alfaro, E. Haplotypes in the CRP Gene Associated with Increased BMI and Levels of CRP in Subjects with Type 2 Diabetes or Obesity from Southwestern Mexico. *Exp. Diabetes Res.* **2012**, *2012*, 982683. [CrossRef]
38. Flores-Alfaro, E.; Fernández-Tilapa, G.; Salazar-Martínez, E.; Cruz, M.; Illades-Aguiar, B.; Parra-Rojas, I. Common variants in the CRP gene are associated with serum C-reactive protein levels and body mass index in healthy individuals in Mexico. *Genet. Mol. Res.* **2012**, *11*, 2258–2267. [CrossRef]
39. Delongui, F.; Lozovoy, M.A.B.; Iriyoda, T.M.V.; Costa, N.T.; Stadtlober, N.P.; Alfieri, D.F.; Flauzino, T.; Dichi, I.; Simão, A.N.C.; Reiche, E.M.V. C-reactive protein +1444CT (rs1130864) genetic polymorphism is associated with the susceptibility to systemic lupus erythematosus and C-reactive protein levels. *Clin. Rheumatol.* **2017**, *36*, 1779–1788. [CrossRef]
40. Enocsson, H.; Gullstrand, B.; Eloranta, M.-L.; Wetterö, J.; Leonard, D.; Rönnblom, L.; Bengtsson, A.A.; Sjöwall, C. C-Reactive Protein Levels in Systemic Lupus Erythematosus Are Modulated by the Interferon Gene Signature and CRP Gene Polymorphism rs1205. *Front. Immunol.* **2021**, *11*, 622326. [CrossRef]
41. Hage, F.G.; Szalai, A.J. C-Reactive Protein Gene Polymorphisms, C-Reactive Protein Blood Levels, and Cardiovascular Disease Risk. *J. Am. Coll. Cardiol.* **2007**, *50*, 1115–1122. [CrossRef]
42. Li, W.; Li, H.; Song, W.; Hu, Y.; Liu, Y.; Da, R.; Chen, X.; Li, Y.; Ling, H.; Zhong, Z.; et al. Differential diagnosis of systemic lupus erythematosus and rheumatoid arthritis with complements C3 and C4 and C-reactive protein. *Exp. Ther. Med.* **2013**, *6*, 1271–1276. [CrossRef]
43. Siemons, L.; ten Klooster, P.M.; Vonkeman, H.E.; van Riel, P.L.; Glas, C.A.; van de Laar, M.A. How age and sex affect the erythrocyte sedimentation rate and C-reactive protein in early rheumatoid arthritis. *BMC Musculoskelet. Disord.* **2014**, *15*, 368. [CrossRef] [PubMed]
44. Meza-Meza, M.R.; Vizmanos-Lamotte, B.; Muñoz-Valle, J.F.; Parra-Rojas, I.; Garaulet, M.; Campos-López, B.; Montoya-Buelna, M.; Cerpa-Cruz, S.; Martínez-López, E.; Oregon-Romero, E.; et al. Relationship of Excess Weight with Clinical Activity and Dietary Intake Deficiencies in Systemic Lupus Erythematosus Patients. *Nutrients* **2019**, *11*, 2683. [CrossRef] [PubMed]
45. Caprio, V.; Badimon, L.; Di Napoli, M.; Fang, W.-H.; Ferris, G.R.; Guo, B.; Iemma, R.S.; Liu, D.; Zeinolabediny, Y.; Slevin, M. pCRP-mCRP Dissociation Mechanisms as Potential Targets for the Development of Small-Molecule Anti-Inflammatory Chemotherapeutics. *Front. Immunol.* **2018**, *9*, 1089. [CrossRef]
46. Chirco, K.R.; Potempa, L.A. C-Reactive Protein as a Mediator of Complement Activation and Inflammatory Signaling in Age-Related Macular Degeneration. *Front. Immunol.* **2018**, *9*, 539. [CrossRef] [PubMed]
47. Shapouri-Moghaddam, A.; Mohammadian, S.; Vazini, H.; Taghadosi, M.; Esmaeili, S.; Mardani, F.; Seifi, B.; Mohammadi, A.; Afshari, J.T.; Sahebkar, A. Macrophage plasticity, polarization, and function in health and disease. *J. Cell. Physiol.* **2018**, *233*, 6425–6440. [CrossRef] [PubMed]
48. Black, S.; Kushner, I.; Samols, D. C-reactive Protein. *J. Biol. Chem.* **2004**, *279*, 48487–48490. [CrossRef]
49. Potempa, L.A.; Rajab, I.M.; Olson, M.E.; Hart, P.C. C-Reactive Protein and Cancer: Interpreting the Differential Bioactivities of Its Pentameric and Monomeric, Modified Isoforms. *Front. Immunol.* **2021**, *12*, 744129. [CrossRef]

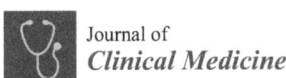

Journal of
Clinical Medicine

Article

C-Reactive Protein (CRP) Blocks the Desensitization of Agonistic Stimulated G Protein Coupled Receptors (GPCRs) in Neonatal Rat Cardiomyocytes

Gerd Wallukat [1], Stephan Mattecka [2], Katrin Wenzel [1], Wieland Schrödl [3], Birgit Vogt [2], Patrizia Brunner [2], Ahmed Sheriff [2,4] and Rudolf Kunze [2,*]

1. Berlin Cures GmbH, BBB Campus, 13125 Berlin, Germany; gwalluk@berlincures.de (G.W.); kwenzel@berlincures.de (K.W.)
2. Pentracor GmbH, 16761 Hennigsdorf, Germany; mattecka@pentracor.de (S.M.); vogt@pentracor.de (B.V.); brunner@pentracor.de (P.B.); ahmed.sheriff@charite.de (A.S.)
3. Institute of Bacteriology and Mycology Faculty of Veterinary Medicine, University of Leipzig, 04103 Leipzig, Germany; schroedl@rz.uni-leipzig.de
4. Division of Gastroenterology, Infectiology and Rheumatology, Medical Department, Charité University Medicine, 12200 Berlin, Germany
* Correspondence: rudolf.kunze@gmx.de

Abstract: Recently, C-reactive protein (CRP) was shown to affect intracellular calcium signaling and blood pressure in vitro and in vivo, respectively. The aim of the present study was to further investigate if a direct effect on G-protein coupled receptor (GPCR) signaling by CRP can be observed by using CRP in combination with different GPCR agonists on spontaneously beating cultured neonatal rat cardiomyocytes. All used agonists (isoprenaline, clenbuterol, phenylephrine, angiotensin II and endothelin 1) affected the beat rate of cardiomyocytes significantly and after washing them out and re-stimulation the cells developed a pronounced desensitization of the corresponding receptors. CRP did not affect the basal beating-rate nor the initial increase/decrease in beat-rate triggered by different agonists. However, CRP co-incubated cells did not exhibit desensitization of the respective GPCRs after the stimulation with the different agonists. This lack of desensitization was independent of the GPCR type, but it was dependent on the CRP concentration. Therefore, CRP interferes with the desensitization of GPCRs and has to be considered as a novel regulator of adrenergic, angiotensin-1 and endothelin receptors.

Keywords: C-reactive protein; adrenergic receptor; desensitization; GPCR signaling; endothelin

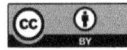

1. Introduction

The homopentameric C-reactive protein (CRP) is a classic acute phase protein that has been known in human medicine for decades. It has been established primarily as a biomarker for active and chronic inflammation of bacterial origin [1] This picture has changed fundamentally. In the 1990s, CRP was identified as a risk factor for atherosclerosis. Relatively low blood levels at >2 mg/L CRP are associated with an increased risk of heart attack, stroke, diabetes and mortality depending on the concentration that was observed [2–4]. Acute inflammation caused by vessel occlusions can be observed in acute myocardial infarction, with rapidly increasing CRP levels up to >100 mg/L over 2–4 days. Restrictions of organic functions may be the consequences of CRP mediated ischemic processes [5,6].

Publications in recent years showed that CRP is more than a biomarker and affects both physiological and pathological processes [5,7–9]. The direct influence of CRP on the cardiovascular system of rabbits has been reported recently [10]. Here, the infusion of human CRP led to a sharp drop in blood pressure within seconds, while the heart rate was not affected. The authors also investigated the influence of CRP on calcium signaling in vitro in two epithelial cell lines. The activation of the cells by adrenoceptor agonists led to intracellular Ca^{2+} mobilization, which was further increased in the presence of CRP [10].

CRP progressively emerges as a molecule with regulatory properties besides its role as an acute phase molecule. In the case of acute inflammation and the associated high CRP levels in the bloodstream, this pentamer primarily has contact with mobile leukocytes and sessile cells lining the vessels, especially endothelial cells. Although interaction with receptors on these cells seems obvious, CRPs molecular action has so far only been investigated on, e.g., Fc receptor γRII (FcγRII) and in the context of macrophage activation and its role as an archaic antibody-like molecule [11–13]. However, one of the fundamental roles of receptor signaling in endothelial cells is the regulation of circulatory parameters, which is mainly mediated by G protein-coupled receptors (GPCRs), specifically adrenergic receptors, angiotensin-II receptor (AT1) and endothelin receptors (ETRs) [14]. Moreover, this is of great impact during excessive inflammatory states, such as, e.g., septic shock, in which circulating CRP levels are dramatically high and hemodynamic parameters are considerably unstable [15,16].

In this respect, it is obvious to examine the influence of CRP on receptor-controlled cell-physiological activation processes. In this paper, we report on the influence of CRP on the signaling system of selected GPCRs, which are involved in the regulation of cardiac, smooth or skeletal muscle cells.

GPCRs are a large group of membrane-bound proteins, the amino acid chain of which crosses the cell membrane seven times. The group is named after the receptor activation triggered extracellularly by agonists, which leads to an interaction with G proteins intracellularly [17]. Adrenoceptors can be classified into five groups (α1, α2 and β1, β2, β3) and are expressed more or less in different tissues and organs of the body [18,19]. They are primarily activated by catecholamines and generally affect the contraction of smooth muscle cells, thereby fundamentally regulating the heart rate and blood pressure. Physiologically important agonists are noradrenaline or adrenaline. Pharmacological, synthetic receptor-specific agonists, such as isoprenaline (β1 and β2-adrenoceptor), clenbuterol (β2-adrenoceptor) or phenylephrine (α1-adrenoceptor), are drugs that are frequently used in pharmacological experiments [14,19,20]. In addition, the peptide hormones endothelin 1 or angiotensin II activate the endothelin ETA and ETB-receptor and the angiotensin II AT1 and AT2-receptor, respectively.

The β1-adrenoceptor is the major adrenergic receptor of the myocardium. Besides this receptor, the β2 and β3 adrenoceptors and the α1-adrenergic, angiotensin II AT1- and endothelin 1 ETA receptors are also expressed in this organ. This receptor expression can be modulated by a long-term treatment with the corresponding agonist and antagonists and also by the agonistic autoantibodies [21–24].

The AT1-, ETA- and α1 receptors are receptors of the blood vessels and are known as vasoconstrictors [25]. However, other receptors such as the β2 adrenoceptor are also expressed in the vasculature. Our investigation has shown that cultured rat cardiomyocytes express a multitude of different G-protein coupled receptors that are coupled to different signal cascades and can change the beating rate of the used spontaneously beating cardiomyocytes [26].

The physiological effect of receptor agonists has been studied for decades on the cultures of neonatal rat cardiomyocytes. These cells beat spontaneously in culture and the change in the pulsation rate after the addition of the agonists can be measured visually on an inverted microscope. This bioassay is a standard cell biological method for the identification and characterization of functional autoantibodies against GPCR or the effect of pharmacological receptor antagonists [27,28].

The aim of the study was to investigate if the inflammatory acute phase protein CRP interferes with the regulation of GPCRs on the cellular level. Here we present first observations about the inhibition of the elementary process of receptor desensitization in rat cardiomyocytes.

2. Materials and Methods

2.1. Pharmacological Agonists and CRP

Human CRP (Pentracor, Hennigsdorf, Germany) was purified from human pooled plasma with a selective CRP-binding matrix as described elsewhere in detail [10]. Endotoxin contamination was avoided, and CRP was stored in its native, pentameric form.

The murine monoclonal antibody (0.64 mg/mL) against CRP was provided by Biometec Inc. (Dr. S. Witt, Biometec GmbH, Greifswald, Germany) and generated by Dr. B. Micheel and Dr. W. Schroedl.

The pharmacological agonists were purchased from Sigma, Germany (Isoprenaline, Phenlyephrine, Endothelin 1, Clenbuterol) or MP Biomedicals, Germany (Angiotensin II) and used in concentrations indicated in Table 1.

Table 1. Effect of CRP on the beating rate of neonatal rat cardiomyocytes stimulated with agonists against GPCRs. The data show the increase or decrease in the beating rate as mean ± standard deviation of the rat cardiomyocytes.

Agonist	n	CRP (50 µg/mL)	Difference in Beating Rate/15 s at Incubation Time (min)				p-Value
			5	120	125	130	130 min, ±CRP
Isoprenaline (1 µM)	5	−	11.76 ± 1.46	9.31 ± 2.07	0.71 ± 0.56	3.47 ± 0.63	<0.001
	5	+	11.26 ± 1.10	11.99 ± 1.66	0.19 ± 0.61	9.91 ± 1.46	
Clenbuterol (3 µM)	4	−	10.69 ± 0.84	7.47 ± 1.93	0.56 ± 0.57	2.58 ± 0.50	0.001
	4	+	10.40 ± 0.91	11.12 ± 0.85	0.28 ± 0.44	9.42 ± 1.33	
Phenylephrine (10 µM)	3	−	7.85 ± 0.81	5.68 ± 1.38	−0.32 ± 0.43	2.84 ± 0.75	0.006
	3	+	7.82 ± 0.51	7.88 ± 0.63	−0.27 ± 0.17	6.89 ± 0.34	
Angiotensin II (1 µM)	3	−	6.11 ± 0.75	3.83 ± 1.16	0.11 ± 0.44	2.17 ± 0.54	0.006
	3	+	5.39 ± 0.61	5.56 ± 0.42	−0.06 ± 0.08	5.17 ± 0.59	
Endothelin 1 (0,1 µM)	4	−	−7.20 ± 0.55	−4.08 ± 1.91	−0.52 ± 0.53	−2.01 ± 0.53	0.002
	3	+	−7.42 ± 0.96	−7.02 ± 0.60	−0.83 ± 0.24	−7.69 ± 0.76	

2.2. Cardiomyocyte Bioassay

The cardiomyocyte bioassay was carried out on neonatal rat cardiomyocytes in cell culture as described elsewhere in detail [27]. Briefly, cardiac myocytes were prepared from heart ventricles of 1–2-day-old Sprague-Dawley rats and cultured in SM20-I medium (Biochrom, Berlin, Germany) with supplemented penicillin (Heyl, Berlin, Germany), heat-inactivated 10% neonatal calf serum (Gibco, Life Technologies, Bleiswijk, The Netherlands), glutamine (Serva, Heidelberg, Germany), streptomycin (HEFA Pharma; Werne, Germany), hydrocortisone (Merck, Darmstadt, Germany) and fluorodeoxyuridine (Serva, Heidelberg, Germany). After seeding the cardiomyocytes with a field density of 160,000 cells/cm^2, the culture medium was renewed after 24 h. The cells were cultured for 2–4 days at 37 °C before using them in the experiment. Target point was the beating rate for 15 s of 6–10 synchronously contracting cell clusters per flask, placed on a heated stage of an inverted microscope at 37 °C. First, the basal beating rate of the cardiomyocytes was measured and after this the agonists were added. The difference between the basal beating rate and increase or decrease in the beating rate after the addition of the agonists is expressed as Δ beating rate/15 s. Respective agonists were then added to the cell culture medium and beating rate was measured again after 5 and 120 min. This was followed by a change of medium (washing 3 times with warm PBS (without calcium), then adding fresh prewarmed (37 °C) complete SM20 culture medium. Thereafter, the pulsation rate returned to the initial value (measured at t = 125 min). After this the stimulation with the agonists was repeated in the same agonist concentration.

For CRP co-incubated cells, human CRP was added in a final concentration of either 50 µg/mL or in decreasing concentrations of 40, 20, 10, 5 and 2 µg/mL and preincubated 10 min before agonist stimulation. CRP was not added again after 125 min.

To block the activity of CRP, it was pretreated with a blocking monoclonal antibody (0.64 mg/mL) directed against CRP for 30 min at room temperature. This mixture was added to the cardiomyocytes like the CRP solution as described above.

3. Results

First, cardiomyocytes were stimulated with isoprenaline (ISO) with and without CRP for 120 min. As expected, ISO increased the beating frequency compared to the basal rate (0; Figure 1A). The initial beating rate was not affected by CRP addition (5 min). After 120 min, cells were washed and the beating rates returned to their basal rate (Figure 1A, 125 min). Then, cells were stimulated again with ISO. In control cells (without CRP), the increase in the pulsation rate was clearly diminished after the renewed stimulation with ISO (Figure 1A, 130 min). This can be explained by the desensitization of adrenergic receptors and was expected [29]. However, with additional CRP incubation, the cardiomyocyte beating rate increased to a similar level compared to the initial stimulation and was significantly higher compared to the control experiment. No desensitization of the response was visible in CRP co-incubated cells. Cells that were treated with CRP preincubated with a monoclonal antibody (mAb) to inhibit the CRP action showed normal desensitization and a beating rate comparable to that in ISO stimulated cells alone after 130 min (Figure 1A). Further, this blocking of the desensitization was concentration dependent. CRP was applied in decreasing final concentrations (40–2 µg/mL) and the same experimental setup was repeated. CRP blocked desensitization after 2nd ISO stimulation in a concentration dependent manner (Figure 1B).

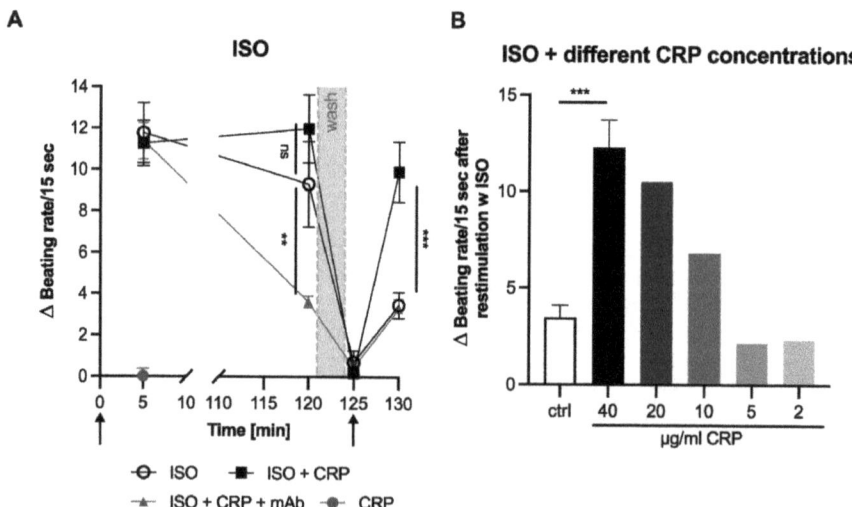

Figure 1. CRP blocks the desensitization of stimulated neonatal rat cardiomyocytes with ISO. Difference of cardiomyocyte beating rates [Δ Beating rate/15 s] modulated by adrenoceptor agonist isoprenaline (ISO) with or without CRP co-incubation. (**A**) Mean of 3–7 independent experiments ± standard deviation is depicted. Arrows indicate stimulation with respective agonists. Grey area indicates washing step. After the washing step, the agonist was added again but no CRP. To test if CRP itself influences the beating rate, cells were incubated with CRP and no change could be observed after 5 min (grey circle). Significance of difference between CRP incubated and control group and mAb group at 120 min and 130 min was calculated with two-way ANOVA with Bonferroni post-hoc test. (**B**) Same experimental setup as depicted in (**A**), but only the beating rate at the last time point (130 min) is shown as mean of 3–5 independent experiments ± standard deviation or as single value (20–2 µg/mL CRP). Significance of difference between 40 µg/mL CRP and control (only ISO) was calculated with student's t-test. ** $p < 0.01$. *** $p < 0.001$. ns: not significant.

This CRP-induced prevention of desensitization was not only seen for the β-adrenoceptors but also for other GPCRs. In our experiments, we additionally tested the effect of CRP on the β2-adrenoceptor (stimulated with clenbuterol (CLE)), the α1-adrenoceptor (stimulated with phenylephrine (PHE)), and the angiotensin II AT1 receptor (stimulated with angiotensin II (ANG)). These receptor agonists also exert a positive chronotropic response and the desensitization of these GPCR was also prevented by CRP (Figure 2). Although phenylephrine and angiotensin II are not highly specific for the indicated receptors, the response can be attributed to these. Only blocking with specific antagonists against these receptors inhibits the chronotropic response in the bioassay [30,31].

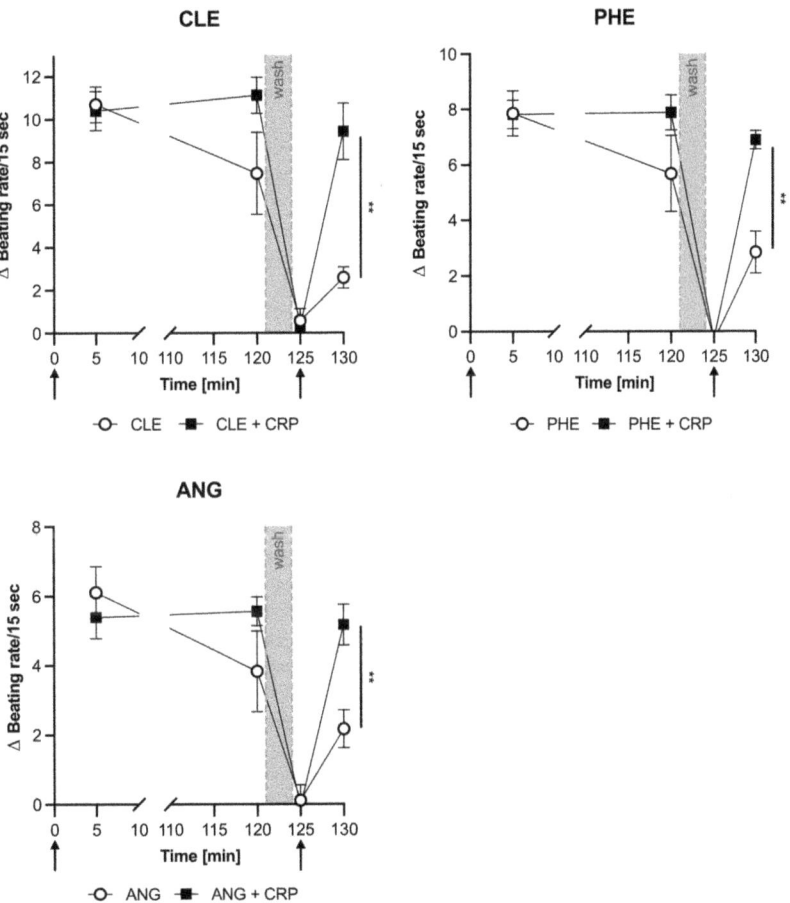

Figure 2. CRP blocks the desensitization of stimulated neonatal rat cardiomyocytes. Difference of cardiomyocyte beating rates [Δ Beating rate/15 s] modulated by agonists clenbuterol (CLE), phenylephrine (PHE) and angiotensin II (ANG) with or without CRP co-incubation. Mean of 3–5 independent experiments ± standard deviation is depicted. Arrows indicate stimulation with respective agonists. Grey area indicates washing step. After the washing step, the agonist was added again but no CRP. Significance of difference between CRP incubated and control group at the last time point was calculated with student's t-test. ** $p < 0.01$.

To investigate whether this was exclusive to positive chronotropic agonists that realize their effects via the α1-, β1-, β2- adrenoceptors or the AT1-receptor, cells were also stimulated with endothelin 1 (ET-1), which binds to ETRs and exerts a negative chronotropic effect in the spontaneously beating rat cardiomyocytes.

ET-1 decreased the cardiomyocyte beating rate initially with and without CRP (Figure 3). Again, responsive receptors were desensitized after 120 min of incubation and after washing and renewed stimulation with ET-1, visible by only slightly decreased beating rates at 120 and 130 min (Figure 3). Co-incubation with CRP abolished the desensitization effect and beating rates were again significantly reduced after renewed ET-1 stimulation.

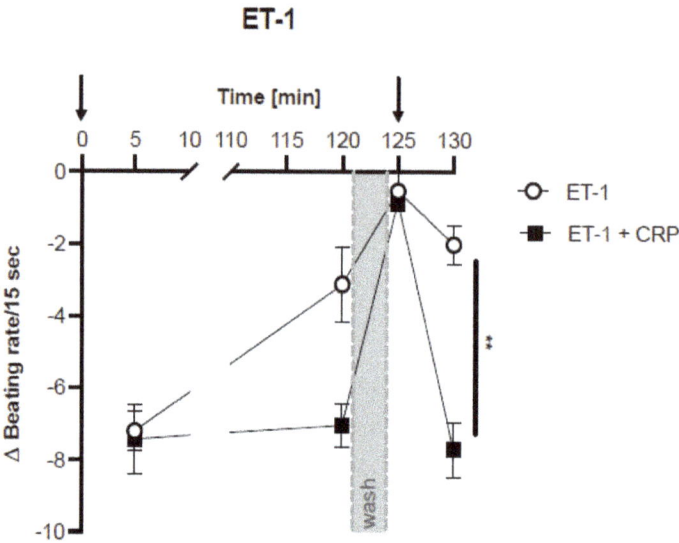

Figure 3. CRP blocks the desensitization of endothelin stimulated neonatal rat cardiomyocytes. Difference of cardiomyocyte beating rates [Δ Beating rate/15 s] modulated by endothelin receptor agonist endothelin 1 (ET−1) with or without CRP co-incubation. ET1 induced a negative chronotropic response. Mean of 4 (control) or 3 (with CRP) independent experiments ± standard deviation is depicted. Arrows indicate stimulation with respective agonists. Grey area indicates washing step. After the washing step, the agonist was added again but no CRP. Significance of difference between CRP incubated and control group at the last time point was calculated with student's t-test. ** $p <$ 0.01.

CRP stimulation alone did not affect the cardiomyocyte beating rate as visible in Figure 1A after 5 min (Δ beating rate/15 s = 0.02 (n = 7)).

Detailed data values of all replicate experiments are listed in Table 1.

4. Discussion

This study was designed to further investigate possible direct effects of CRP on GPCR signaling. Therefore, an established in vitro model was used, spontaneously beating neonatal rat cardiomyocytes, which react to stimulations with agonists or antagonists of different GPCRs with a change of beating rates [32].

Stimulation of cardiomyocytes with different adrenergic, AT-1 and ETR agonists readily affected their beating rate as expected. Co-incubation with CRP did not influence the basal beating rate nor the initial effect of the agonistic stimulation. However, desensitization of GPCRs, which was observed with all used agonists, did not occur in CRP co-incubated cardiomyocytes (Figures 1A, 2 and 3, 130 min). Re-stimulation with either isoprenaline, clenbuterol, phenylephrine, angiotensin or endothelin-1 showed a significant chronotropic effect in CRP co-incubated cells, on a similar level as the initial stimulation. This was already visible as a trend after 120 min, when CRP-co-incubated cells showed slightly higher beating rates than agonist-only treated cells (Figures 1A, 2 and 3, 120 min), albeit not significant. CRP pretreated with a blocking monoclonal antibody, blocked the effect seen in the presence of CRP and led to the desensitization of the receptor-mediated response. Surprisingly, the antibody influenced the beating rate after 120 min and led to a significant reduction compared to cells treated only with isoprenaline or with isoprenaline and CRP (Figure 1A, 120 min). Fetal calf serum has been shown to contain CRP [33]. It cannot be excluded that this already has an effect, although the neonatal calf serum has been heat inactivated. Since CRP was not suspected of influencing this test system, this issue has not yet been investigated.

This leads to the conclusion that this acute phase protein somehow inhibits the mechanism of desensitization. This phenomenon, which is the same in all GPCRs examined, suggests ubiquitous mechanisms that take place via the cell membrane and therefore, potentially affect all GPCRs.

GPCR signaling is naturally regulated in a highly complex manner and on several levels. Desensitization is a basic physiological principle, employed by cells in order to protect themselves from overstimulation and possible exhaustion. Receptors can be rendered unresponsive by sequestering or degrading them or downstream intracellular messengers. Rapid desensitization, which would be the case in our applied experimental timeline, is mainly achieved by GPCR phosphorylation, uncoupling the receptor from its respective G protein [29]. This phosphorylation is mostly mediated by GPCR kinases, leading to binding of arrestins, which block further signaling [34].

The blockade of desensitization of the examined GPCRs achieved by CRP goes beyond the known inflammatory properties of CRP. To hypothesize which molecular route CRP modulates in order to produce a second chronotropic reaction to GPCR agonists would be purely speculative and cannot be deduced from these results. It is, however, in line with previous findings, showing a direct effect of CRP on intracellular calcium signaling, which was further increased by ISO or PE stimulation, no matter the order of stimulation [10]. Interestingly, in this experimental setup, when the used GPCR agonist was washed away after 120 min, CRP in the culture medium was also washed off and not reapplied. Hence, the observed effects stem from the pre-incubation of cells with CRP. This means that either CRP is still bound to the cell membrane after washing or already modulated intracellular components, thereby affecting GPCR desensitization. Although this would be a novel action of CRP, it has been previously reported that CRP can either directly stimulate other receptors than Fcγ on cells [35,36] or regulate their expression in vascular smooth muscle cells [37]. This already indicated that the physiological function of CRP is far more complex than assumed.

Obviously, the protective mechanism of the fast desensitization of GPCRs is inhibited by an elevated level of CRP in vitro, with possible pathophysiological consequences in vivo. Hemodynamic parameters are often unstable in extreme inflammatory settings such as sepsis, which also present dramatically high circulating CRP levels with peaks of $\geq$150 mg/L CRP [15,16]. Although no direct effect of CRP on hemodynamic variables has been shown so far in CRP-infused humans, this is most likely because the published experimental setups have focused on long-term effects or rather low CRP concentrations [38–40]. The recently published results in rabbits [10] are in line with the here described effects, which hint towards a process in which CRP itself affects blood pressure and heart rate by modulating complex GPCR signaling in endothelial cells and/or cardiomyocytes.

In conclusion, the acute phase protein CRP may play an important role in the regulation of GPCR signaling. By blocking the desensitization of different GPCRs, CRP—in combination with the corresponding agonist—induces a permanent receptor stimulation that may represent a dangerous pathogenic factor. This permanent stimulation of cells could induce a calcium overload, apoptosis and subsequent cell death. Investigations could be conducted to determine whether this effect on the GPCR regulation could play an additional role in the context of the CRP-mediated tissue destruction during ischemic processes [5]. Therefore, it may be meaningful to remove the elevated CRP levels not only after myocardial infarction [6] but also in, for example, sepsis.

The findings described herein should be a springboard for more elaborate experiments to characterize and understand the molecular details of CRP-mediated inhibition of GPCR desensitization.

Study Limitations

The studies were carried out on primary neonatal rat cardiomyocytes. Their cell-specific receptor equipment is to be seen primarily as a signaling system. Whether this phenomenon also occurs in other cell types such as endothelial cells was not investigated. Other test systems such as calcium signaling are suitable for this. It should also be a focus to find out more about the molecular mechanism of receptor desensitization including whether CRP directly interacts with the respective GPCRs or other receptors on the cardiomyocytes. If similar data are obtained this way, then the conclusions on the pathophysiological effects of CRP on the homeostasis of GPCR could be further elaborated.

Author Contributions: G.W., W.S., B.V., A.S. and R.K. conceptualized and planned the experiments. G.W. and K.W. performed the experiments. G.W., S.M. and P.B. analyzed the data. P.B., A.S. and R.K. wrote the manuscript. All authors contributed to the article and approved the submitted version. All authors have read and agreed to the published version of the manuscript.

Funding: No funding was received for this research.

Institutional Review Board Statement: Ethical review and approval was not required for the animal study because Isolation of Cardiomyocytes was performed without prior experimental intervention and had to be only reported and not approved by federal agencies. All experiments were performed in accordance with the German law for animal protection.

Informed Consent Statement: Not applicable.

Data Availability Statement: The original contributions presented in the study are included in the article, further inquiries can be directed to the corresponding author.

Conflicts of Interest: S.M. and P.B. are employees of Pentracor GmbH. B.V., A.S. and R.K. are cofounders and shareholders of Pentracor GmbH. A.S. is CEO of Pentracor GmbH.

References

1. Sproston, N.R.; Ashworth, J.J. Role of C-Reactive Protein at Sites of Inflammation and Infection. *Front. Immunol.* **2018**, *9*, 754. [CrossRef]
2. Ridker, P.M.; Everett, B.M.; Thuren, T.; MacFadyen, J.G.; Chang, W.H.; Ballantyne, C.; Fonseca, F.; Nicolau, J.; Koenig, W.; Anker, S.D.; et al. Antiinflammatory Therapy with Canakinumab for Atherosclerotic Disease. *N. Eng. J. Med.* **2017**, *377*, 1119–1131. [CrossRef]
3. Ridker, P.M.; MacFadyen, J.G.; Everett, B.M.; Libby, P.; Thuren, T.; Glynn, R.J.; Group, C.T. Relationship of C-reactive protein reduction to cardiovascular event reduction following treatment with canakinumab: A secondary analysis from the CANTOS randomised controlled trial. *Lancet* **2018**, *391*, 319–328. [CrossRef]
4. Torzewski, J. C-reactive protein and atherogenesis: New insights from established animal models. *Am. J. Pathol.* **2005**, *167*, 923–925. [CrossRef]
5. Sheriff, A.; Kayser, S.; Brunner, P.; Vogt, B. C-Reactive Protein Triggers Cell Death in Ischemic Cells. *Front. Immunol.* **2021**, *12*, 273. [CrossRef]
6. Ries, W.; Torzewski, J.; Heigl, F.; Pfluecke, C.; Kelle, S.; Darius, H.; Ince, H.; Mitzner, S.; Nordbeck, P.; Butter, C.; et al. C-Reactive Protein Apheresis as Anti-inflammatory Therapy in Acute Myocardial Infarction: Results of the CAMI-1 Study. *Front. Cardiovasc. Med.* **2021**, *8*, 155. [CrossRef]
7. Venugopal, S.K.; Devaraj, S.; Yuhanna, I.; Shaul, P.; Jialal, I. Demonstration that C-reactive protein decreases eNOS expression and bioactivity in human aortic endothelial cells. *Circulation* **2002**, *106*, 1439–1441. [CrossRef]
8. Anzai, T.; Yoshikawa, T.; Takahashi, T.; Maekawa, Y.; Okabe, T.; Asakura, Y.; Satoh, T.; Mitamura, H.; Ogawa, S. Early use of beta-blockers is associated with attenuation of serum C-reactive protein elevation and favorable short-term prognosis after acute myocardial infarction. *Cardiology* **2003**, *99*, 47–53. [CrossRef]
9. Jenkins, N.P.; Keevil, B.G.; Hutchinson, I.V.; Brooks, N.H. Beta-blockers are associated with lower C-reactive protein concentrations in patients with coronary artery disease. *Am. J. Med.* **2002**, *112*, 269–274. [CrossRef]

10. Bock, C.; Vogt, B.; Mattecka, S.; Yapici, G.; Brunner, P.; Fimpel, S.; Unger, J.K.; Sheriff, A. C-Reactive Protein Causes Blood Pressure Drop in Rabbits and Induces Intracellular Calcium Signaling. *Front. Immunol.* **2020**, *11*, 1978. [CrossRef]
11. Bharadwaj, D.; Stein, M.P.; Volzer, M.; Mold, C.; Du Clos, T.W. The major receptor for C-reactive protein on leukocytes is fcgamma receptor II. *J. Exp. Med.* **1999**, *190*, 585–590. [CrossRef]
12. Manolov, D.E.; Rocker, C.; Hombach, V.; Nienhaus, G.U.; Torzewski, J. Ultrasensitive confocal fluorescence microscopy of C-reactive protein interacting with FcgammaRIIa. *Arterioscl. Thromb. Vasc. Biol.* **2004**, *24*, 2372–2377. [CrossRef] [PubMed]
13. Kaplan, M.H.; Volanakis, J.E. Interaction of C-reactive protein complexes with the complement system. I. Consumption of human complement associated with the reaction of C-reactive protein with pneumococcal C-polysaccharide and with the choline phosphatides, lecithin and sphingomyelin. *J. Immunol.* **1974**, *112*, 2135–2147.
14. Wang, J.; Gareri, C.; Rockman, H.A. G-Protein Coupled Receptors in Heart Disease. *Circ. Res.* **2018**, *123*, 716–735. [CrossRef] [PubMed]
15. Varpula, M.; Tallgren, M.; Saukkonen, K.; Voipio-Pulkki, L.M.; Pettila, V. Hemodynamic variables related to outcome in septic shock. *Intensive Care Med.* **2005**, *31*, 1066–1071. [CrossRef] [PubMed]
16. Castelli, G.P.; Pognani, C.; Cita, M.; Stuani, A.; Sgarbi, L.; Paladini, R. Procalcitonin, C-reactive protein, white blood cells and SOFA score in ICU: Diagnosis and monitoring of sepsis. *Minerva Anestesiol.* **2006**, *72*, 69–80. [PubMed]
17. Weis, W.I.; Kobilka, B.K. The Molecular Basis of G Protein–Coupled Receptor Activation. *Ann. Rev. Biochem.* **2018**, *87*, 897–919. [CrossRef]
18. Bylund, D.B.; Eikenberg, D.C.; Hieble, J.P.; Langer, S.Z.; Lefkowitz, R.J.; Minneman, K.P.; Molinoff, P.B.; Ruffolo, R.R., Jr.; Trendelenburg, U. International Union of Pharmacology nomenclature of adrenoceptors. *Pharmacol. Rev.* **1994**, *46*, 121–136.
19. Brodde, O.-E. Beta-adrenoceptors in cardiac disease. *Pharmacol. Ther.* **1993**, *60*, 405–430. [CrossRef]
20. Lymperopoulos, A.; Rengo, G.; Koch, W.J. Adrenergic Nervous System in Heart Failure. *Circ. Res.* **2013**, *113*, 739–753. [CrossRef]
21. Podlowski, S.; Luther, H.P.; Morwinski, R.; Muller, J.; Wallukat, G. Agonistic anti-beta1-adrenergic receptor autoantibodies from cardiomyopathy patients reduce the beta1-adrenergic receptor expression in neonatal rat cardiomyocytes. *Circulation* **1998**, *98*, 2470–2476. [CrossRef]
22. Brodde, O.E. Beta 1- and beta 2-adrenoceptors in the human heart: Properties, function, and alterations in chronic heart failure. *Pharmacol. Rev.* **1991**, *43*, 203–242.
23. Brodde, O.E.; Michel, M.C. Adrenergic and muscarinic receptors in the human heart. *Pharmacol. Rev.* **1999**, *51*, 651–690.
24. Wallukat, G. The beta-adrenergic receptors. *Herz* **2002**, *27*, 683–690. [CrossRef]
25. Lukitsch, I.; Kehr, J.; Chaykovska, L.; Wallukat, G.; Nieminen-Kelha, M.; Batuman, V.; Dragun, D.; Gollasch, M. Renal ischemia and transplantation predispose to vascular constriction mediated by angiotensin II type 1 receptor-activating antibodies. *Transplantation* **2012**, *94*, 8–13. [CrossRef]
26. Wallukat, G.; Schimke, I. Agonistic autoantibodies directed against G-protein-coupled receptors and their relationship to cardiovascular diseases. *Semin. Immunopathol.* **2014**, *36*, 351–363. [CrossRef]
27. Hohberger, B.; Kunze, R.; Wallukat, G.; Kara, K.; Mardin, C.Y.; Lammer, R.; Schlotzer-Schrehardt, U.; Hosari, S.; Horn, F.; Munoz, L.; et al. Autoantibodies Activating the beta2-Adrenergic Receptor Characterize Patients With Primary and Secondary Glaucoma. *Front. Immunol.* **2019**, *10*, 2112. [CrossRef]
28. Wenzel, K.; Wallukat, G.; Qadri, F.; Hubner, N.; Schulz, H.; Hummel, O.; Herse, F.; Heuser, A.; Fischer, R.; Heidecke, H.; et al. Alpha1A-adrenergic receptor-directed autoimmunity induces left ventricular damage and diastolic dysfunction in rats. *PLoS ONE* **2010**, *5*, e9409. [CrossRef]
29. Lefkowitz, R.J.; Pitcher, J.; Krueger, K.; Daaka, Y. Mechanisms of β-Adrenergic Receptor Desensitization and Resensitization. In *Advances in Pharmacology*; Goldstein, D.S., Eisenhofer, G., McCarty, R., Eds.; Academic Press: Cambridge, MA, USA, 1997; Volume 42, pp. 416–420.
30. Luther, H.P.; Homuth, V.; Wallukat, G. Alpha 1-adrenergic receptor antibodies in patients with primary hypertension. *Hypertension* **1997**, *29*, 678–682. [CrossRef]
31. Wallukat, G.; Homuth, V.; Fischer, T.; Lindschau, C.; Horstkamp, B.; Jupner, A.; Baur, E.; Nissen, E.; Vetter, K.; Neichel, D.; et al. Patients with preeclampsia develop agonistic autoantibodies against the angiotensin AT1 receptor. *J. Clin. Investig.* **1999**, *103*, 945–952. [CrossRef]
32. Haase, N.; Herse, F.; Spallek, B.; Haase, H.; Morano, I.; Qadri, F.; Szijarto, I.A.; Rohm, I.; Yilmaz, A.; Warrington, J.P.; et al. Amyloid-beta peptides activate alpha1-adrenergic cardiovascular receptors. *Hypertension* **2013**, *62*, 966–972. [CrossRef]
33. Schroedl, W.; Jaekel, L.; Krueger, M. C-reactive protein and antibacterial activity in blood plasma of colostrum-fed calves and the effect of lactulose. *J. Dairy Sci.* **2003**, *86*, 3313–3320. [CrossRef]
34. Gurevich, V.V.; Gurevich, E.V. GPCR Signaling Regulation: The Role of GRKs and Arrestins. *Front. Pharmacol.* **2019**, *10*, 125. [CrossRef] [PubMed]
35. Richter, K.; Sagawe, S.; Hecker, A.; Kullmar, M.; Askevold, I.; Damm, J.; Heldmann, S.; Pohlmann, M.; Ruhrmann, S.; Sander, M.; et al. C-Reactive Protein Stimulates Nicotinic Acetylcholine Receptors to Control ATP-Mediated Monocytic Inflammasome Activation. *Front. Immunol.* **2018**, *9*, 1604. [CrossRef] [PubMed]
36. Meng, S.; Zhang, L.; Zhao, L.; Fang, Y.R.; Fujimoto, T.; Hirano, S.; Inoue, H.; Uchihashi, K.; Nishikawa, Y.; Wu, Y.F. Effects of C-reactive protein on CC chemokine receptor 2-mediated chemotaxis of monocytes. *DNA Cell Biol.* **2012**, *31*, 30–35. [CrossRef] [PubMed]

37. Wang, C.H.; Li, S.H.; Weisel, R.D.; Fedak, P.W.; Dumont, A.S.; Szmitko, P.; Li, R.K.; Mickle, D.A.; Verma, S. C-reactive protein upregulates angiotensin type 1 receptors in vascular smooth muscle. *Circulation* **2003**, *107*, 1783–1790. [CrossRef]
38. Bisoendial, R.J.; Kastelein, J.J.; Levels, J.H.; Zwaginga, J.J.; van den Bogaard, B.; Reitsma, P.H.; Meijers, J.C.; Hartman, D.; Levi, M.; Stroes, E.S. Activation of inflammation and coagulation after infusion of C-reactive protein in humans. *Circ. Res.* **2005**, *96*, 714–716. [CrossRef]
39. Bisoendial, R.; Birjmohun, R.; Keller, T.; van Leuven, S.; Levels, H.; Levi, M.; Kastelein, J.; Stroes, E. In vivo effects of C-reactive protein (CRP)-infusion into humans. *Circ. Res.* **2005**, *97*, e115–e116. [CrossRef]
40. Birjmohun, R.S.; Bisoendial, R.J.; van Leuven, S.I.; Ackermans, M.; Zwinderman, A.; Kastelein, J.J.; Stroes, E.S.; Sauerwein, H.P. A single bolus infusion of C-reactive protein increases gluconeogenesis and plasma glucose concentration in humans. *Metabolism* **2007**, *56*, 1576–1582. [CrossRef]

MDPI
St. Alban-Anlage 66
4052 Basel
Switzerland
www.mdpi.com

Journal of Clinical Medicine Editorial Office
E-mail: jcm@mdpi.com
www.mdpi.com/journal/jcm

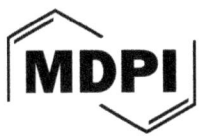

Disclaimer/Publisher's Note: The statements, opinions and data contained in all publications are solely those of the individual author(s) and contributor(s) and not of MDPI and/or the editor(s). MDPI and/or the editor(s) disclaim responsibility for any injury to people or property resulting from any ideas, methods, instructions or products referred to in the content.